Over
Addiction

CORINNE SWEET

Overcoming Addiction

Positive steps for
breaking free of addiction
and building self-esteem

PIATKUS

TO

CLARA LUCY SWEET

My Grandma,
first friend and playmate

© 1994 Corinne Sweet

First published in 1994 by
Judy Piatkus (Publishers) Ltd of
5 Windmill Street, London W1P 1HF
www.piatkus.co.uk

This revised and updated edition published in 1999

The moral right of the author has been asserted

*A catalogue record for this book is
available from the British Library*

ISBN 0-7499-2015-7 pbk

Designed by Chris Warner
Illustrations by Chartwell Illustrators

Set in Linotron Baskerville
by Computerset, Harmondsworth, Middlesex
Printed and bound in Great Britain by
Butler & Tanner Ltd, Frome, Somerset

Acknowledgements

Thanks to my literary agent Carole Blake of Blake Friedmann and Melissa Harrison at Piatkus Books for getting this new edition into print.

Heartfelt love and thanks to Rufus Potter for continued understanding and patience and to Clara Potter-Sweet for inspiration and fun. Thanks also to Corinne Haynes, Hayley Baker, Marika Denton and Margaret Evans for invaluable practical support.

Thanks, too, to the many counselling clients and interviewees who were prepared to reveal and learn from their pain.

Finally, thanks to Jo and the late Leslie Sweet, without whom this book would not have been possible.

Contents

'One must have chaos in oneself in order to give birth to a dancing star'

FRIEDRICH NIETZSCHE

Preface to the New Edition

As the 20th Century gives way to the new Millennium, with all its promise and challenge, many of us are still held back by the myriad ways in which we continue to hurt ourselves in everyday life. Addiction remains one of those thorny issues that still seems to confuse and scare. Pessimists believe addiction is part of the human condition and will never be 'cured' except through constant abstinence and vigilance.

I disagree. I believe that our propensity to hurt ourselves through everyday chemical and emotional addictions is only a measure of how we have been hurt when young and growing. As we become more conscious and aware as a society and as individuals about how and why these hurts occur – and as we learn more about recovering from them successfully – there is every reason to be optimistic.

Addiction is an Achilles heel for anyone who has been unloved, abused, hurt, disliked, isolated or punished as a child. The increased publicity about such mistreatment, and how to heal it, has been a major step in the direction of healing our culture and ourselves. I don't believe things are getting worse, I just think things are becoming more open, more talked about.

And as people become aware of what has happened to them it becomes possible to make choices. It's entirely possible to choose living healthily and positively over living unhealthily and self-destructively. It takes time, honesty and effort, but it is entirely possible to overcome addiction. Sometimes we need to get help with the process from healers, therapists, counsellors or self-help groups, but this is usually an extremely positive step.

Of course, there will be slip-ups, mistakes and discomfort on the way, but the outcome can be so rewarding and fulfilling that chemical and emotional addictions simply erode. If you can be your own best friend, love yourself completely and learn to choose positive options, rather than negative ones, then addiction will have no further place in your life.

Overcoming addiction is a process, not an instantaneous quick fix. But I believe it is entirely possible and desirable to treat yourself in the best way possible to get the most out of your one, precious life.

Corinne Sweet,
March 1999

Introduction

You've picked up this book and started reading for a reason.

Maybe you have an inkling that you're hooked on something like cigarettes, eat too many sweets or are simply fed up having the same old repetitive, dead-end relationships?

It might be you've recently begun to realize, much to your intense discomfort (perhaps after seeing a TV programme, reading a magazine article or talking to a friend), that you could be addicted to something serious, such as alcohol or tranquillizers, which is beginning to threaten your health, work, social and family life. So you've probably been scouring bookshops for more information and help.

You might have been struggling with one particular addiction for several years – caught in a cycle of giving up and starting again – and feel hopeless you'll ever crack it.

Maybe you want to help someone you love or care for because you think they're addicted and heading for trouble?

You might already have succeeded in giving up a major addiction, such as smoking or over-eating, and you now want to tackle another, say, overworking or caffeine.

Perhaps you're just curious about the subject?

Whatever your motive for reading, you're going to feel a wide range of emotions just opening this book. The word 'addiction' is very loaded. It usually brings up an image of a scrawny heroin addict or meths-downing dosser, wallowing amid filthy needles and general squalor – certainly nothing to do with you.

You may well be reading this book with some trepidation, eager to reassure yourself that you're all right (Phew! – I'm not really addicted, so I can carry on as usual). Or you might be looking for evidence to *confirm* your worst fears – that you *are* addicted, so you can frighten yourself into doing something about it.

You might even have the urge to slam this book shut and chuck it in the bin, shouting 'rubbish' (this can also be a sign that a raw nerve has been struck). You may even feel so uneasy that you have to rush off and make a soothing cup of coffee or down a comforting glass of wine; light up a steadying cigarette or turn on the TV to blot out what the book's brought up to the surface for you.

Rest assured – these are completely normal reactions to looking at anything to do with addiction. Many of us feel frightened by imagining life without our regular, everyday props. Habits and rituals provide a reassuring framework in an uncertain world. However, if your habits harm you in any way, you may well be reading this book to find out if there's any alternative.

NEW PERSPECTIVE

On this more positive note, this book might bring you some relief. It may help that someone understands your private struggles. Its aim is to empower you, to remind you of any previous successes you've had in giving up your addictions and help you pinpoint what you can do not only to overcome your addictions but stay off for life. It is about having a chance to look at your life from a completely new perspective. It may be comforting that something that's been lurking in the back of your mind is finally being acknowledged and explained. More importantly, if you persevere with reading this book, you should learn what you yourself can do about your everyday addictions.

Part One: Becoming Addicted looks at the reasons for addiction and helps you identify if you're hooked. It also covers facing and releasing the feelings underlying your addictions, with the aim of helping you to give up self-abuse forever.

Part Two: Overcoming Addiction explains how you can give up your chemical and emotional addictions by being your own parent and nourishing yourself by meeting your emotional, physical, sexual, social, creative, intellectual and spiritual needs instead.

Part Three: Staying Off for Life explains how to live positively by getting ongoing support, improving your health and working out a lifeplan while learning to play, relax and enjoy yourself.

Throughout the book you will find lots of blocks of questions for you to answer. These are designed to help you set down your own feelings about the various topics covered, and if you answer them honestly they will gradually build up into an encouraging record of your progress.

Because you may well prefer to keep this record completely private, I suggest that you set aside a special notebook (a 'reporter's pad' is useful) for this purpose. You don't need to copy out all the questions laboriously first. Simply start each block of answers on a fresh sheet, writing down the relevant book page number at the top for ease of reference, and then setting down the number of each question with your answer alongside. It will then be just a matter of placing your note-book answers alongside the relevant page whenever you want to review or update what you have recorded. And your privacy will be assured.

Part One

——◦——

Becoming Addicted

Chapter 1

———■○■———

Are You Addicted?

Thirteen people are perched on chairs in a circle looking like a bomb is about to drop. When I enter the room, some flinch visibly, some look away, some smile nervously, and one reaches for a cigarette – it may be her last, so she's damned well going to smoke it in defiance of 'teacher'. All are clasping mugs of tea and coffee. Two seats are empty, awaiting the inevitable late-comers.

WELCOME TO THE WORKSHOP

There are always one or two people who find it impossible to get to a 'giving up addictions' workshop, even if they've paid the full fee. When the morning of the workshop comes, terror grips their hearts and it's definitely safer to snuggle under the duvet and drift back to sleep. Those boring household chores suddenly seem enormously seductive and, frankly, *anything* would seem better than having to think about giving up addictions.

But there are always those – and today there are 13 – who have decided that it is time for a change. Some people come out of simple curiosity or because they have a nagging feeling that they might be addicted to something. Often, they are at a significant crossroad in their lives, such as a relationship splitting up, having a baby, starting a new career, losing a job,

7

being made redundant, children leaving home, reaching a certain age, say, 21, 40 or 60, getting ill or recovering from a serious illness, retiring, wanting to lose weight, cut down drinking or give up smoking. And it is usually because they are fed-up with being ruled by self-destructive habits. Today, these 13 brave souls are shivering on their seats, wondering what unpleasant thing is going to happen next.

Within half an hour the group's mood has changed beyond recognition. The relief is tangible, and audible. The room is filled with laughter and cheers, shoulders have dropped, bags and mugs are no longer clutched, arms are no longer folded in defence. There is almost a party atmosphere. I always set a tone of 'cheerful boasting' at the start. It never fails to work. This allows people to 'own up' to their everyday addictions in a confidential, non-judgemental atmosphere. It also counteracts any shame and embarrassment they may feel.

No-one is told off or disapproved of, no-one is made to feel weird or excessive. Everyone gets to relax and laugh as the truth about their addictions is welcomed. I encourage group members to cheer each other on, literally. It is a major relief for people to get the chance to proclaim what they do to themselves in a supportive environment.

Ruth, a large white woman in her forties, stands up, her knees knocking, her hands trembling. 'Well, I have to admit I over-eat.' (Cheers from the group.) 'I love chocolate, biscuits, cakes, ice cream (cheers) and I especially love eating at night (hooray). I also drink too much wine (cheers) and I pick my spots.' (Applause.)

Ruth sits down proudly. Next comes Mo, a young black woman. 'I spend far too much money on clothes (cheers). In fact, I spend too much altogether (loud cheers). I smoke dope every weekend (hooray), and I drink coffee till it comes out of my ears.' (Wild applause).

Mo giggles shyly as she sits. There is a pause while the group finishes clapping, then Peter, a tall, middle-aged white man, gathers himself up to his 6ft and says with a mischievous grin, 'I steal and I gamble (muted cheers).' He pauses, looks around and then clears his throat. 'I also go to bed with a different woman every week (whoops and applause), and I drink too much whisky and beer (applause).'

And so it goes on until each member of the group has 'owned up' to their own particular everyday addictions. As the group continues going round, each person's individual list gets longer as they discover addictions they never realized they had. There's a lot of: 'oh, I never thought of that as an addiction before – I'm addicted, too!' By the end of this ice-breaking exercise there is a general realization that there's a lot of defensiveness about 'owning up' to addictions and people are tangibly relieved to find they have got so much in common. Because of this, their sense of isolation begins to lessen from this point.

LOW SELF-ESTEEM

Addictions are built on a vicious cycle of low self-esteem: You have addictions because you feel bad about yourself, and you don't like yourself because you're addicted. People are usually shy and embarrassed about 'owning up' to something they're not proud of doing to themselves. They say they feel ashamed, guilty, humiliated about their everyday addictions (that's why people with addictions usually underestimate or deny what they're doing when quizzed). Intuitively, deep down, we know we're harming ourselves, even if we laughingly call it 'over-indulgence' or 'a bit of fun'. If you don't like yourself much, or even hate yourself, then you will not really care what you do to yourself. You may even be doing it to punish yourself. If you accept bad treatment as normal, then your everyday addictions are a way of continuing that mis-treatment. So low self-esteem goes hand in hand with addictions and any steps you take towards living addiction-free must necessarily be based on building your self-esteem.

At workshops I ask people early on what they love about themselves and I am quite often met with silence, tears, embarrassment, anger, laughter and meek statements like 'my eyes are quite nice', or 'I suppose I'm quite a kind person'. It is very hard for people to evaluate themselves accurately or positively, because they have so often been put down for being 'big-headed', or for 'showing off' and 'blowing their own trumpet'. Learning to like, even love, yourself is crucial for giving up addictions – yet people can find it more excruciating to identify three things they like about themselves than to carry on hurting themselves instead. However, if people begin to see themselves in a more positive light, the ball starts rolling inexorably towards overcoming their addictions.

SUCCESS BREEDS SUCCESS

I always focus on successes people have had in giving up addictions to date – no matter how trivial. It is much easier to put yourself down for what you haven't done, rather than remember what you have already achieved. Group members work in pairs to list what they have already tried to cut down, give up, or have conquered totally. This exercise is essential for confidence-building, as nothing breeds success like success.

Review Your Own Successes

So, before we go any further, why not take a moment to stop and think about *your* own successes in giving up your addictions so far. You will find it very useful to write down all your answers to the following questions in a notebook, so that as you work through this book you build up your own private record. See the Introduction for full details.

1. Have you ever cut down an addiction before? If yes, which and when?

   ....

2. How did you do it?

   ....

3. If you slipped back into the addiction – what situation triggered it off again? And was your addiction less pronounced? The same? Worse?

....

4. Have you ever succeeded in giving up an addiction (or any addictions) completely? If yes, which? How long ago?

....

5. If you have succeeded completely, how many attempts did it take to give up finally. What did you learn about yourself? (for example that you're anxious or find it hard to relax, or that you're shy and use your addictions for 'Dutch courage'.)

....

Even if you have tried to give up an addiction one, two, 12 or 20 times – and have not yet succeeded fully – **give yourself a pat on the back**. Few people ever give up any addiction after one attempt. It can take many attempts, many months or even years, plus many different methods, before an addiction is finally cracked.

Yet each time you try to give up an addiction, you are taking a step in the right direction. Even continuing to read this book is another step towards final success. Just keep reminding yourself of what you have already achieved. Copy out the list of what you have already given up (if you have), and stick it on a wall in your bathroom, bedroom or on your fridge or mirror. Write it in your diary – and look at it often. Give yourself credit on daily, weekly, monthly, yearly anniversaries. It's a great way of cheering yourself on.

HOW ADDICTED ARE YOU?

For this book to be of use, you need to find out what, if anything, you're addicted to, and how much. Try answering the following quiz as honestly as you can (you may feel you want to skip over these pages and leave some questions out, or to be economical with the truth.) **Remember: this quiz is for your eyes only.** You don't have to tell anyone else about it. Write down your answers in your notebook, as before. Remember to start a fresh page.

	Yes	No

1. Do you *have* to have a cup of tea or coffee to get you going in the morning?

2. Do you drink more than four cups of tea or coffee a day?

3. Do you smoke cigarettes?
   If yes, do you smoke: between 1 and 10 a day? between 10 and 20 a day? over 20 a day?
   ....

4. If you smoke, do you smoke more when you drink alcohol socially?

5. Do you use (soft) illegal drugs, such as cannabis?
   If yes, do you use them: daily? once a week? seldom?
   ....

6. Do you use (hard) illegal drugs, such as cocaine, ecstasy, heroin, or crack?
   If yes, do you take them: daily? weekly? occasionally?
   ....

7. Do you drink alcohol?
   If yes, do you drink: daily? weekly? monthly? occasionally?
   ....

8. Do you drink alcohol alone?

Yes No

9. Do you get drunk?
   If yes, do you get drunk: regularly?
   infrequently?

   ....

10. Do you have memory blanks?

11. Would it seem impossible for you to have a
    social life or a celebration without alcohol?

12. Do you take tranquillizers, anti-depressants
    or sleeping pills?
    If yes, do you take them: regularly?
    occasionally? Also do you fear living without
    them?

    ....

13. Do you watch TV?
    If yes, do you watch it: daily? once a week?
    occasionally?

    ....

14. Do you watch anything that happens to be
    on?

15. Do you have sex?
    If yes, do you feel you have to have it: more
    than once a day? daily? twice a week?
    weekly? occasionally?

    ....

16. Do you masturbate?
    If yes, do you feel you have to do it: more
    than once a day? daily? weekly? occasionally?

    ....

17. Do you fantasize in order to have an orgasm?

18. Do you use pornography in your sex life?

19. Do you go out and spend money to cheer
    yourself up?

Yes   No

20. Do you fear opening your bank statements?

21. Do you fall in love frequently?

22. Do you distract yourself with an addictive habit when you get upset?

23. Do you fear strong feelings – either in others or yourself?

24. Are you constantly on a diet or watching your weight?

25. Do you eat more, and even binge, when you are unhappy, scared and lonely?

26. Do you stop eating altogether when you are upset?

27. Do you sometimes get urges to hurt yourself?
If yes, have you ever slashed, bruised or injured yourself?

28. Do you daydream and find reality frightening?

29. Do you feel people who don't drink, smoke, take drugs, etc, are rigid and boring?

30. Do you have relationships which seem to end up the same old way, time after time (i.e. you get left when you get too attached, or you leave when it gets too serious?)

31. Do you feel you couldn't cope without your favourite, everyday addictions?

The above quiz is designed to help you to identify your addictions for yourself. Look at your answers. The more 'yes' answers you have, the more your life is based on everyday addictions. Look at what the answers show you about yourself. What have you owned up to which you hadn't thought of as an

14

addiction before? Only you know the truth about what you do to yourself, so if you've cheated in the quiz, you've cheated yourself.

You might feel worried that you suddenly seem to have so many addictions. And you might be surprised that things like TV, masturbation and sex are included. After all, these are likely to feature on everyone's lists. But what you have recorded regarding frequency will begin to give you some idea whether you are addicted or not. This book is designed to give you insights, information and practical advice to help you get yourself off the hook – *but only if you want to.*

WHAT IS AN ADDICTION?

In general, an addiction is a habit or behaviour which is:

- Not under your control – rather *it* controls you. You feel you have no choice but to do it, take it, behave like it. Once addicted, you're on automatic pilot.

- A compulsion, so entrenched in your daily life, such an unthinking habit, that you hardly recognize that you're doing it (and if people point it out you get defensive, angry, irritable, feel secretive, deny it, get a 'sinking feeling', etc).

- Something you do over and over and over, more and more and more for a bigger and better 'hit', 'thrill', or 'kick'.

- Something you turn to regularly, when you want to numb out unpleasant feelings like boredom, loneliness, frustration, exhaustion, sadness, anger, unhappiness, physical pain, rejection, jealousy, self-loathing, failure.

- Something which feels life-threatening to do without; you feel you simply couldn't cope without it.

- Time-consuming. You can spend a lot of your life struggling with whether to cut down, give up, or keep off your addictions.

- Self-obsessive. You can waste a lot of precious emotional and mental energy agonizing about your addictions, hiding, handling and struggling against them.

- A drain on your resources. Either you spend a lot of money on them and/or put valuable time and energy into them (and recovering from the self-abuse created by them), to the detriment of more positive things in your life.

- Probably sapping your power. Reducing your effectiveness, your self-esteem, disrupting your family, social, love and work life, while damaging your physical and mental health.

In excess, addiction can ruin and endanger lives – even kill.

The Addictive Trap

At workshops I always describe addictions as being like leeches – sticking to your body, sucking the life-blood out of you, reducing your power, refusing to be winkled off, except by direct means. Once an addiction has got a grip it will fight to the death before letting go. Of course, you may fear that you would fall apart completely without such props. Reacting strongly to the question, 'What would life be like without your favourite addictions?', people can get defensive, tearful or even storm out.

Rebecca, a bright Australian musician in her thirties, told one workshop group, 'I'd go completely berserk if I didn't have my afternoon shot of sugar. Around three or four every day I get a craving and I have to rush out and buy masses of cakes, biscuits, chocolate, anything sweet. I'm a raving, bad-tempered witch without sugar. I just couldn't imagine my life without it and don't you damn well tell me I've got to give it up.' Rebecca was red-faced, sweating and shaking with fear by the time she got to the end of this speech. Just telling us about her sugar addiction was enough for her to feel threatened. Of course, nobody in the group, including myself, was going to force her to do anything or tell her off – that would neither be appropriate nor effective.

The problem with any addiction, is that it can keep you trapped by limiting your freedom and putting you at the mercy of a self-destructive habit. Rebecca wanted to lose weight, spend less money, get fit, make friends. Instead, she regularly bought and binged on excessive amounts of sweet foods and afterwards felt miserable, sordid and very alone. Although she was fearful and angry about 'owning up' to us, she became visibly relieved when she was accepted wholeheartedly. She burst into tears and sobbed like a small, helpless child in the arms of a neighbour. I kept reassuring her that it was fine to cry, that she was releasing old pain, and was safe and respected for showing her feelings.

Rebecca poured out her grief for a full 15 minutes, and went on crying on and off for the rest of the day. At the end of the workshop, she said she felt immensely relieved, especially because a whole façade of secret isolation had begun to be chipped away. It was Rebecca's first step towards overcoming her sugar addiction. (For more on isolation, see Chapter 2: Facing and Releasing Emotions and Chapter 8: Making the Break.)

Chemical Addictions

When we think of the word 'addiction' we nearly always think of the chemicals that we can get hooked on. And we usually believe that if we give up, hey presto, we'll no longer be addicted.

This is obviously a very simplistic view. For instance, if you're regularly consuming vast amounts of alcohol it would definitely be a good idea to stop drinking so heavily or, better still, take a break altogether. However, it *is* possible for someone to stop drinking and yet still be what is called a 'dry alcoholic' – because the painful emotions which drove them to seek relief in alcohol have not been dealt with. Until that is done the addicted person remains hooked emotionally, even if no longer actively destroying their body with alcohol. And if the underlying emotional patterns stay intact, there is a serious risk that another addiction will quickly take its place – smoking, mind-changing drugs, over-eating, workaholism – or that they may return to alcohol later on.

When we think of chemical addictions, we tend to think of the most popular ones: tobacco, alcohol, tranquillizers and caffeine. Here's a longer list of chemical addictions people have identified at my workshops, and in counselling sessions:

- Alcohol
- Tea
- Coffee
- Cola and caffeine, sugar and additive-loaded fizzy drinks
- Sugar
- Chocolate
- Food
- Peanuts
- Salt
- Smoking
- Alka-Seltzer
- Marijuana
- Ecstasy
- LSD
- Cocaine
- Heroin
- Magic mushrooms
- Anti-depressants
- Tranquillizers
- Sleeping pills
- Analgesics (pain killers)
- Slimming pills
- Glue
- Petrol
- Amyl nitrate ('poppers')
- Laxatives

Are there any more you can add from your own experience? Write them down in your notebook.

....
....

Emotional Addictions

Over the past few years there has been a growing awareness among health professionals, psychologists, counsellors and, indeed, people trying to give up addictions, that not only are most addictions psychologically as well as physically addictive, but also there are addictions which seem to be purely what I call 'emotional addictions'. People use their emotional addictions in the same way they use a substance, the only difference being that they have an addiction to a repetitive, self-abusive form of *behaviour* (which may or may not include the use of chemicals).

Here is a list of emotional addictions people have identified at my workshops and in counselling sessions:

- Compulsive starving (Anorexia).
- Compulsive eating ('bingeing'), followed by self-induced vomiting (bulimia).
- Compulsive eating without vomiting.
- Junk food.
- Overworking (workaholism).
- Excessive sport and fitness training.
- Pornography (and masturbating with pornography).
- Falling in love repeatedly, even when emotion is not reciprocated.
- Falling in love with 'bastards'.
- Compulsive masturbation.
- Compulsive caring (also called Codependency).
- Self-mutilation.
- Picking scabs/spots/sores.
- Scratching.
- Biting nails/skin.
- Make-Up.
- Looking immaculate all the time; looking in mirrors.
- Compulsive house-cleaning every day (or night).
- Hoarding money.
- Compulsive spending/shopping (credit cards, etc).
- Playing video games.
- Gambling/playing fruit machines.
- Stealing.
- Telling lies.
- Pretending.
- Day dreaming, fantasizing.
- Sexual fantasies.
- Compulsive sex.
- Compulsive celibacy.
- Sado-masochism.
- Watching/listening to soap operas.
- Getting ill.
- Exhaustion.
- Being a victim/martyr.
- Telephone calls.
- Sleeping.
- Hurrying, being busy, busy, busy.
- Compulsive radio listening.
- Compulsive TV/video watching.
- Violence.
- Junk reading (bonkbusters, comics, etc).
- Driving too fast.
- Danger, taking risks, thrills.
- Procrastination.
- Shutting people out.
- Being miserable.
- Continually complaining, grumbling, etc.
- Compulsive reading.

Are there any more you can add from your own experience? Write them down in your notebook.

....

....

Overlapping Addictions

Although I usually make a distinction between chemical and emotional addictions, there is an obvious overlap. Eating disorders are a good example. Some people are addicted both to the chemicals in food, such as sugar, caffeine, additives, and also to what food represents or reminds them of psychologically, becoming an emotional comforter or anaesthetic.

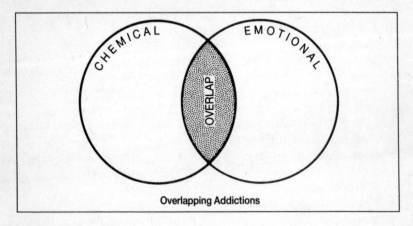

Overlapping Addictions

You may think that some of the above addictions, such as being 'busy, busy, busy' or being miserable, are not addictions and that I'm stretching the concept too far. I encourage people to define for themselves what their emotional addictions are, from the perspective that *it is a behaviour which they use to blot out painful reality, which they repeat endlessly, and about which they feel guilty, powerless and/or sordid.*

For instance, 'busy, busy, busy' people are hurling themselves into frenzied activity to stop themselves feeling their feelings. They are usually driven by fear (of death, disease, failure . . .), to be hyperactive and avoid intimate relationships. Similarly, people addicted to being miserable may know, intuitively, that this is a misguided way of trying to get attention for past hurts. It is misguided because, as we shall see in Chapter 2, trying to compensate in the present for past pain never works. We can only grieve and come to terms with what we never had or have lost.

Multiple Addictions

From my counselling work, and my own experience, it seems to me that our lives are often constructed on a fine, interwoven fabric of 'uppers' and 'downers' to keep ourselves going. In other words, most of us have multiple addictions. We need caffeine and sugar to help us get up (early morning tea and coffee, sugary breakfasts – sugar-laden cereals, jam/honey/ marmalade, etc); have 'elevenses' for a 'pep up' and caffeine drinks to keep going, spend money to feel better, masturbate or have sex to relax and to stop feeling lonely; and alcohol, sleeping pills, excessive TV/video watching, use of pornography and so on to 'wind down' or 'blank out'.

TRIGGERS

One addiction can trigger another. Petra, a young, unemployed woman wrote to me in despair about her compulsive sexual behaviour, which was linked to drinking alcohol. 'For me, ending up in bed with strange men is *always* tied to alcohol,' she wrote. 'I can't sleep with someone without a fair bit to drink – then I can pick up a man, *any* man. The trouble is, I can't foresee a future without alcohol or men – and I couldn't cope at all without both.' Petra knew already that drinking lowered her inhibitions and allowed her to act on her compulsion for sex (and that compulsion was due to feeling bad about herself while desperately wanting to feel better). 'It was only when I became pregnant by one of ten different men, all total strangers, that I thought I'd better stop.'

Stopping drinking (and not going out to pubs and bars), meant Petra didn't need to act on a compulsion to pick up men once drunk. She began to see one addictive behaviour (drinking), would inevitably 'trigger' the other (picking up men and having sex with them). Once she had understood this, she realized she needed to tackle the emotional problems underlying her addictions, if she was to free herself from both, permanently.

KNOWLEDGE IS POWER

Once you become aware, like Petra, that your emotional and chemical addictions overlap, such as being nervous about making a phone call and lighting a cigarette; having an alcoholic drink when you're under pressure or bored; or going out on a spending-spree when premenstrual or lonely); then you need to take radical steps to give up your addictions because they harm you. Knowledge is power.

You also need to recognize what feelings and moods tend to trigger you to act addictively. Are you feeling irritable, frustrated, bored, lonely, angry, unhappy when you reach for your comforters? (For further explanation see Chapter 2).

Ask yourself right now, which of the addictions you wrote on your list trigger other addictions? Write them down in your notebook in pairs. (For example, watching TV leads to eating chocolate, drinking alcohol socially leads to smoking, feeling lonely leads to food bingeing).

....

....

TACKLING ADDICTIONS

You need to be honest with yourself when you look at your addictions, though it might take some time before you can face the whole truth – because many of us are in what is called 'denial'. This means that it's too uncomfortable to face reality, so you deny it to yourself. If past experiences have been too painful, or even life-threatening, we protect ourselves psychologically by burying these memories. This is especially true of traumas in early life, when you were completely dependent on other people for safety, nourishment, care, and love. This means that we often only start remembering and/or recognizing the significance of these traumas in later life, once we are adults, capable of surviving independently. However, denial can occur at any age.

Consequently, it is very hard to know whether you are 'in denial' or not, *because when you're in denial, you don't know you're in denial, because you're in denial!* If you give up your addictions, however, hidden memories and feelings begin to emerge. This means you could well begin to remember painful or upsetting incidents. This might sound off-putting, and not like a benefit at all, but many people experience immense relief as these memories begin to help them to understand what the root causes of their addictions are. In particular, they are helped to stop blaming themselves for being 'bad' or 'weak-willed'. As you, too, will learn as you begin to exorcise the hurts underlying an addiction, it will cease to run your life.

That is why I set up workshops and counselling sessions on addiction with firm rules about confidentiality. As you saw at the beginning of this chapter, it is crucial not to be judgemental or moralistic, but rather to allow people plenty of time and loving encouragement to own up and define their addictions for themselves. People need correct information, caring, uncritical attention, plus loving support to 'come out'. This provides the safety to own up to the truth, cast off 'denial' and begin to get a sense of their real selves.

Turning Points

You will probably only ever be motivated enough to give something up once you have seen how harmful, humiliating, even degrading your addictions are to you. These flashes of insight create a 'turning point' – the moment at which you decide to get off the hook and start afresh.

One woman told me about waking up after a night's heavy drinking to find vomit in her wastepaper basket. She was horrified. It was clearly hers, but she had no memory of vomiting and suddenly she was scared, not only by the alcohol-induced memory blank, but also by the fact that she could have died by choking in bed. This was the turning point for her; she decided from that moment to stop drinking.

Another example was a man who waited all day in the rain to meet his heroin dealer. After six hours he suddenly saw himself, waiting for his fix like a dependent bedraggled dog. This was his turning point: his humiliation and degradation enabled him to walk away without drugs and seek help.

You may think that these alcohol and heroin-dependent people have nothing to do with you, but they do. All addiction operates in a similar way, whether your 'fix' is chocolate or cocaine. Only the *degree of harm* is at issue. Often, only by going to the very edge of your endurance do you begin to want to overcome your addiction.

'Tweezer Movement'

If you assume that there are emotional reasons for your addiction, be it Mars bars or compulsive gambling, then it's helpful to adopt what I call the 'tweezer movement' – whereby you tackle your addiction from two sides at once. For instance, Petra realized she needed to employ the tweezer movement of giving up alcohol (her chemical addiction) which triggered having compulsive sex (her emotional addiction). Petra also had to decide not to pick up men (emotional addiction again) and drinking to get 'Dutch courage' (chemical addiction).

Adopting the tweezer movement means: giving up the chemical addiction which is probably numbing, damaging, even destroying your brain, body and life. Without tackling this head on there is little chance of your being able to think about real alternatives. By withdrawing from your fix, you will soon begin to understand more about the distresses you've been repressing, because they will probably start bubbling up to the surface – you will *feel* more. I'll be discussing this in detail in Chapter 2.

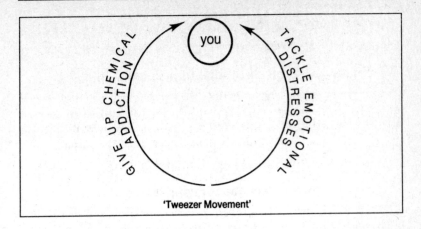

'Tweezer Movement'

Then you need to tackle the emotional distresses underlying the urge to numb out and harm yourself. For instance, think about a main chemical addiction that you may already have identified and want to give up. Try answering these questions in your notebook:

1. When did it start?

....

2. Where did you learn this addictive behaviour?

....

3. Who/what initiated you?

....

4. What did it mean to you at the time?

....

5. Was it a pleasant or unpleasant experience?

....

6. What was going on in your life at the time?

....

7. What role did it play?

....

8. What were your real needs then?

....

9. What were you feeling at the time?

....

10. Do you still need to do it now (or is it just habitual)?

....

11. How would you feel about giving it up?

....

12. Have you ever substituted this addiction with another? If yes, which, how and when?

....

DEALING WITH THE WORST FIRST

It obviously makes sense to tackle the worst, possibly life-threatening, addictions first. People often come to me worried about their eating and then, during a counselling session, reveal that they smoke or drink excessively. It can seem easier to face the less life-threatening addictions first, because you feel you would fall apart completely without your major addiction to, say, nicotine or alcohol. Obviously, some chemical addictions are more harmful than others. It would be ridiculous to say, for instance, that sugar is as harmful as heroin, or LSD is less harmful than TV-watching – though they all perform the same task of blurring or blotting out reality.

SUBSTITUTION

If you do not deal with the underlying distresses of a chemical and/or an emotional addiction, you can tend to substitute one addiction for another when you try to give up. You might stop smoking and start eating more sweets, or stop drinking alcohol and drink pints of tea, instead. You have to guard against a tendency to blot out feelings, using anything that comes to hand or mind. The most important thing is to recognize what you do to yourself and understand your 'triggers'. Then you can start tackling your addictions with the tweezer movement, dealing with the most life-threatening addiction(s) first.

CODEPENDENCY

A word of warning. If you are reading this book to assess whether someone you are close to is addicted – you may well have a problem yourself – *of being hooked on helping those close to you*. This is called codependency, and is usually a way of not facing up to your own emotional difficulties. As long as your partner, mother, child, boss, or friend is the person with a problem, you can feel useful, worthwhile and normal in relation to them. In fact, it is a way of trying to control other people and your relationships with them. It may be well-meaning, but it is often misguided and can be the cause of much bitterness and resentment. You can't live other peoples' lives for them – nor should you ever try to. So if you think you are reading this book for this purpose, you might find it helpful to read *Codependency: How to Break Free and Live Your Own Life* by David Stafford and Liz Hodgkinson (see 'Help' section).

SELF-HELP IS BEST

Nobody can ever get anyone else to give up an addiction successfully. It only works if you are ready and willing to overcome them for yourself. All the nagging, cajoling, emotional blackmailing, or bullying in the world, will only serve to worsen an existing relationship. You probably already know that you'll only do something when *you* want to. Being pushed by someone else can cause you to get stubborn, to rebel, take revenge, pretend, lie or withdraw. Even if you feel it is a sign of someone caring about you when they push you to give up an addiction, their caring can feel claustrophobic. If their love is conditional upon your doing what they want, that can make you feel manipulated and trapped.

If this is your feeling, you might need to look at why you let other people boss you around. Is that the only way you can feel cared for? Is it because you find it hard to take responsibility for your own life? Whatever the reason, only YOU can decide to give up an addiction FOR YOURSELF. Helping yourself for yourself is the only motivation that works long-term.

ASSESSING YOUR PRIORITIES

To reiterate: you can only really start overcoming your addictions once you've acknowledged you have them – and that's why it is essential to face up to what you're hooked on. It may be a quite straightforward addiction (or addictions), which can be easily handled. Or you may feel that you need urgent attention (if this is so, turn to the 'Help' section at the back of the book).

Keeping this in mind, go back to the quiz on page 12 and remind yourself how you scored. Then look at the list of chemical and emotional addictions (on pages 18 and 19) as well as those you wrote down in your notebook yourself.

Now ask yourself and write down you answers in your notebook:

1. Which addiction could I definitely not bear to give up (or even think about giving up)?

....

2. If you know you are addicted to several things and you know that one or two are more harmful, or even life-threatening, than the others, write them down in your notebook, in order of priority. Put the most serious at the top and the least serious at the bottom. Begin with the words:

My addictions, in order of seriousness, are:

....

Pat yourself on the back: By admitting what you do to yourself, you have just taken the first step towards overcoming your addictions. You may feel the urge to ditch this book right now, because it all feels 'too much'. Don't; you are probably just feeling scared – which is natural. What follows in the rest of the book will help you get off the hook – **if you want to.**

The next step is to understand why you have addictions, what they do to you and how they're sustained. Understanding a problem is a necessary part of solving it, so it is important for you to see that your addictions actually hold you back in life, instead of helping you (which is the illusion most of us cling on to – 'I couldn't go to that job interview without having a stiff drink and a cigarette first').

Chapter 2

———— o ————

Facing and Releasing Your Emotions

When I first started giving up my own addictions 20 years ago, I was terrified of unleashing a deluge of pent-up feelings. How would I cope without cigarettes to push down my fear before facing difficult situations or people? How would I manage my physical pain from a serious road accident without numbing out on alcohol, painkillers and drugs? How would I deal with my loneliness and lack of self-esteem if I ceased to throw myself into endless romantic and sexual encounters? How would I get through each day without endless mugs of coffee and tea to pep me up?

FEAR OF LOSING CONTROL

I feared being engulfed by unpleasant emotions and, especially, losing control. I was very skilled at hiding my real feelings in those days. No matter how bad I felt inside, I always managed to be the scintillating 'life-and-soul' of any party. I listened to people for hours as they confided about their problems, and I seldom talked about mine. I overworked all the time and ignored my physical well-being. I was terrified of letting my drug-induced mask slip. Deep inside, I was desperately longing to talk about myself, be understood, loved, cared for and accepted. Instead, I propped myself up daily on 'uppers' and 'downers' so I could go to work, do the house chores, have relationships – but all at one remove. Nobody got to see the real, vulnerable, sensitive and needy me. In fact, I was petrified they would, because I felt inside that I was pretty worthless, unlovable, even wicked. I can now look back at those periods of my teen and young adult life with wonder at the massive strain it was to keep everything bottled up. It is like viewing the Dark Ages through the thin end of a telescope.

Today, I am no longer frightened of facing and releasing my feelings and am much better at recognizing my emotional states. This includes moods which could lead me to act self-destructively through addictions. I no longer fight them, I'm not desperate to mask them from my friends and work colleagues, and I have learned what is appropriate to show and tell. Most of all, I have accepted my feelings as part of me, an essential element in being alive, and I know I need to face and release my feelings on a regular basis to be healthy, productive and balanced. I no longer trust what makes me 'feel good' as the guide to what actually *does* me good.

And it's increasingly socially acceptable to be fully feeling human beings. As we learn more about psychology and physiology, the old divisions between body, mind and spirit are narrowing. We understand a lot more about how emotions affect health (via the immune system): how having a good cry, a good laugh, or a shout, can make us much more mentally and physically healthy. We are becoming aware of the need to unbutton the top collar, unstiffen the upper lip – and let rip. We go to sporting events to shout, pop events and fun-fairs to scream, horror films to shake, romantic movies to cry and comedy shows to laugh. Nationally broadcast disasters like Hillsborough, Zeebrugge, King's Cross and the Marchioness, have taught us that it's vital to spend time recovering emotionally as well as physically. Yet even though we may know more about what we need emotionally we can still be shy about asking for it directly, not wanting to be vulnerable or needy by showing how we really feel.

The 'Feel Good Factor'

One of the most confusing things about addictions is that, for a time, they can make you feel relaxed, euphoric, carefree, happy and powerful. That is what I call the 'Feel Good Factor'. At workshops, people say, 'But if I like to drink, and it makes me feel good, why should I give it up?'

The answer is this: things that make you 'feel good' are not necessarily good for you. (And things that are good for you do not necessarily make you feel good – in the short term at least.) So, if an addictive substance or behaviour makes you feel good, that is not necessarily a true measure of what it is doing for or to you. You need to look at the long-term results rather than the short-term 'highs' or instant effects. Alcohol, cocaine and compulsive sex can make you 'feel good' in the short-term, but they are not necessarily good for you in the long-term, especially if you feel they are the *only* things that make you feel good, fully alive or give your life meaning.

Isolation and Disconnection

Isolation is the key to addictions. That feeling of deep-down loneliness, of being misunderstood, not belonging, not being cared for or listened to, of being unimportant, stems from the experience of being left in emotional pain. Ironically, it is something we all have in common (if only we realized it). Many of us are disconnected from ourselves, not knowing how we really feel or what we want at any given moment. Disconnection can be dangerous, because it may lead you to do something self-abusive, or hurtful to others, simply because you're so 'out of touch' with yourself.

Remember, as we saw in Chapter 1, addictions:

- Are based on and reinforce feelings of low self esteem: you are not worth anything, so it doesn't really matter if you abuse yourself.

- Numb you out and stop you feeling uncomfortable, scary and painful feelings.

- Distort reality and give you an illusion of being in charge when you're not.

- Harm you – physically, psychologically, emotionally.

- Limit your personal, professional and social powers.

- Make you 'feel good' while masking your real feelings.

- Keep you disconnected from yourself.

The phoney 'feel good' sense of happiness, well-being, satisfaction, euphoria, always wears off in time, leaving you feeling flat, bored, lonely, depressed, irritable, hung over, miserable, broke, sordid, and worse. Then you need to re-enact the addiction to get 'up' again, which is inevitably followed by another 'down'. The underlying feelings are not really 'magicked away' by feeling good using an addictive substance or behaviour. In fact, it can result in making you feel twice as bad as before, because coming down to earth can feel a lot harder once you have been up in the clouds.

THE ADDICTIVE TREADMILL

I call this 'up' and 'down' cycle the 'Addictive Treadmill'. You no longer control your addictions – they control you. Once you are hooked on to it, it can govern your life.

How the Addictive Treadmill works:

1. You are feeling bad (whether you know it consciously or not): fed-up, bored, shy, isolated, frightened, sad, rejected, angry, a failure, unloved. Or you are feeling under pressure and need to relax, forget and unwind. So you turn to your favourite addiction for relief.

2. You get some relief. You 'feel good' for a while: minutes, hours, even days. You get a feeling you can cope or relax because the addiction has numbed out and masked your

real underlying feelings. Under the influence you might take risks, act irrationally, make bad decisions or procrastinate – but why give a damn? You feel good, you only have one life and, you argue, why not live it to the full?

3. You come down – usually with a bang. Ouch! All the problems and difficulties you tried to escape from are still there. And now you also feel tired, flat, irritable, exhausted, disappointed, rejected, sordid, physically ill and/or angry from having acted addictively. You have probably spent too much money, wasted time, got into tangles with people, said/done things you regret, got behind at work. You feel wretched and full of self loathing. You want to blame someone or something, you want to cover up the fact you went over-the-top (you probably pretend nothing happened). You are secretly scared (but would never admit it). You feel bad-tempered and let-down, even suicidal sometimes. You hate feeling like this, you want to 'feel good' again, and quickly. And you know what makes you feel good in the short-term. Your favourite addictions, so . . .

4. You act addictively again, only this time you need a bigger dose to cover up your initial bad feelings PLUS the bad feelings from having just acted addictively PLUS the knowledge you're acting addictively again to cover it all up . . .

So round and round and round and round you go on the Addictive Treadmill.

The Addictive Treadmill usually escalates until it collapses, with you under it. Maybe you have a crisis, such as getting ill, losing your job, running out of credit, failing an exam, getting arrested, rowing with a good friend, breaking up with a lover or missing a deadline. Whatever, something traumatic usually happens which forces you to stop, feel and think.

It is hard to get off the Addictive Treadmill once you're on it, because the feelings bubbling away under the surface can feel very threatening to face. You would probably rather die than face them head on. In order to be able to step off the Addictive Treadmill voluntarily, you have to understand why you have such feelings in the first place. That you need to learn to live with and handle them, instead of fearing them and desperately trying to escape.

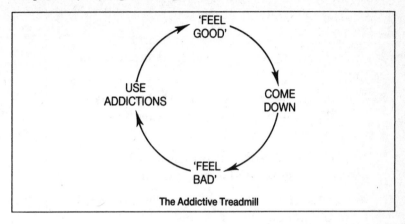

The Addictive Treadmill

HOW WELL DO YOU KNOW YOUR EMOTIONS?

Try doing this quiz by ticking either yes or no to the following questions. Or write down the question numbers and your yes/no response in your notebook.

Yes   No

1. Do you feel worried about what this quiz might reveal?

2. Do you ever feel unattractive and unlovable?

3. Do you ever feel numb and just want to blank out?

4. Do you find it hard to let yourself cry?

5. Do you find it difficult to cry with other people?

Yes No

6. Do you sometimes get swamped with feelings of self-loathing and believe you're deeply bad, damaged, etc.?

7. Do you often feel alone, separate and different from other people (and superior or inferior, or both)?

8. Do you have delayed reactions to things (like critical comments), only feeling hurt hours, days or weeks after the event?

9. Do you find it hard to express yourself directly to people and avoid confrontation?

10. Are you secretive, hiding things you do even from the people closest to you?

11. Do you swing between going over the top and being very self-controlled?

12. Are you often fearful, frustrated, angry, but bottle it all up and then explode?

13. Do you feel pessimistic, fearing the worst so you won't be disappointed?

14. Do you find it hard to trust people?

15. Are you frightened about people knowing the 'real you'?

16. Do you sometimes feel empty or hollow inside and desperately need something to fill the gap?

17. Do you lose your temper at the wrong time and in the wrong place?

18. Do you find it hard to tell if people like you?

19. Do you worry a lot?

20. Do you know when you're happy?

Yes No

21. Do you think women are 'more emotional'
than men?

Scoring

Count up your 'yes' answers.

1–7 'yes' answers: you may be fairly unaware of your
emotions, or denying how you really feel. Go through the
answers you said 'no' to and double check how you really feel.
What do your 'yes' answers tell you, about you?

8–15 'yes' answers: you're probably fairly aware of your
feelings and are quite a balanced person. Look again at your
'no' answers – double check them and notice which they were.
What do they tell you about you?

16–21 'yes' answers: you're very aware of your feelings,
perhaps over-analytical and even quite anxious as a person.
Are there any 'yes' answers you'd say 'no' to on second
thoughts?

1. How did you feel doing the quiz? Take a moment just to
consider how you felt – write it down in your notebook.
....

2. Also, write down how you feel now you know your score.
....

3. What do you know about yourself that you didn't know
before?
....

EMOTIONAL LITERACY

We don't get any formal training in understanding our
emotions, yet the whole of our lives we need to be able to

communicate and relate to people at home, at work, on the
street – in fact, everywhere. This process, of learning to
recognize, face and handle your own feelings, I call 'emotional
literacy'. Of course, the more your understand your own
feelings,the better you can empathize with other people's.

As a culture, we meet our need for emotional literacy by
consuming vast quantities of TV and radio soap-operas,
novels, newspapers and magazines, which provide an endless
diet of problems (rape, abortion, death, marriage, separation,
illness, child sexual abuse, bankruptcy, alcoholism, accidents,
unemployment, drug-addiction, sexual harassment, racism)
and their apparent solutions. Eager for information, millions
of people perch on the edges of their seats every day, watching
the TV screen to see men crying, women raging, children
fighting back, in the quest for greater understanding and
control over their own lives.

Women's magazines (especially the ever-popular 'Agony
Aunt' columns) are a valuable source of emotional literacy. A
granny wrote to *Woman* magazine: 'I'm such an emotional
person, I cry at soaps on television, at books and even at the
verses inside greetings cards! It's so embarrassing . . . is there
anything I can take to help myself?' The idea that she should
'take something' (probably a tranquillizer) shows how terrified
people can be of completely natural emotional expression.

When new clients come to see me, I spend the first few
sessions reassuring them that emotions are completely
acceptable. As their emotions start to surface, they usually
apologize for crying, getting angry or being fearful and
mistrusting and feeling very embarrassed, humiliated and
shy. They cover their faces with their hands, swallow back tears
and suppress their shakes. There is always a lot of fear about
'losing control'. All those booming voices from childhood:
sneering siblings, censorious school-teachers, punishing
parents, are still shouting 'grow up', 'cry baby' or 'pull yourself
together', in their heads. But with encouragement people can
soon begin to accept, recognize and release their feelings in a
safe environment. They can learn pretty quickly that there is
really nothing to fear. We are usually more frightened of fear,

than of what caused the fear itself; emotions are emotions – that's all.

Why You Have Emotions

Emotions are a natural and essential part of being human, they are not just annoying things that get in the way of your having a smooth, trouble-free life. Emotions have a purpose, they:

- Help you to react to, connect with and love other human beings.

- Warn you of danger and help you to survive.

- Enable you to reproduce and nurture the human species in a complex environment.

- Provide a channel for experiencing and assessing that environment.

- And most of all, provide a means of healing emotional hurts.

'Good' and 'Bad' Emotions

We can all experience a wide range of emotions, from dark despair to jubilant euphoria. However, as a culture, we've tended to label some emotions as 'good', and therefore acceptable, and others as 'bad', and therefore unacceptable. For instance, we tend to think of emotions as polar opposites:

'Good' Emotions	'Bad' Emotions
Love	Hate
Connectedness	Isolation
Affection	Aggression
Happiness	Unhappiness
Excitement	Fear
Passion	Boredom
Sexual arousal/desire	Frigidity
Generosity	Jealousy/Envy/Greed
Contentment	Irritability

Satisfaction	Dissatisfaction
Energy	Exhaustion
Serenity	Desperation

Some people become 'sunk' in negative emotions and cannot believe there are any positive emotions to experience. This can leave many feeling 'bad' and/or depressed, with a deep sense of failure and chronic mistrust. Others are permanently proving how positive they are and fear facing the darker side of their emotions because they would no longer 'feel good'. However, it is possible and necessary for mental and physical health to find a balance between positive and negative emotions. (See also Chapter 10: Meeting Your Emotional Needs.)

Moods

We usually refer to our good and bad emotions as 'moods'. We say 'I'm in a filthy mood', or 'He's in a great mood, today'. These are very non-specific descriptions of a wide spectrum of feelings. Really, they only denote whether you feel 'up' or 'down'. Mostly, we accept this as a rough guide in everyday life, but few of us ever delve any deeper. At addictions workshops I ask people 'how do you feel?' and I am usually met with a look of confusion or a simple answer of 'fine' or 'OK'. With further probing, I usually get nearer the truth. When I ask private clients how they are feeling, they will say 'All right', even when I can see they are really feeling sad, angry or afraid.

Of course, you can't spend the whole of your life describing in minute detail to everyone you meet how you are – that would be absurd. But fewer misunderstandings, rows, accidents, mistakes and unhappiness would occur if we were trained to be more aware of our feelings, how we communicate them through moods and how these moods impact on those around us.

In addition, men are particularly hampered by having to be 'cool' and 'tough' at all costs, which means they can be very unaware of their emotional states. Women, on the other hand, are thought of traditionally as 'too emotional'.

Being Upset

Another short-hand term is 'being upset'. This can mean anything from being miserable to furious. As we saw above, few of us are really attuned to our feelings finely enough to know how we feel at any moment. It is often only people in the caring professions, such as social workers, counsellors, healers, doctors, and therapists; or artists, such as actors, writers and poets; or people in recovery from addiction of various types, who have learned to tune in to their moods and can recognize their feelings accurately. In fact, it's often disparaged as being very 'American' or 'navel gazing' to spend too much time analysing your feelings. But, if you want to get off the hook from your everyday addictions, a necessary step will be to learn about emotions and, in particular, to become familiar with your own emotional repertoire.

FACING YOUR EMOTIONS

Here are some more questions for you to answer in your notebook.

1. Are there any emotions you fear facing? If yes, write them down.

   ....

2. Why do you fear them?

   ....

3. Are there any emotions you fear facing in others? If yes, write them down.

   ....

4. Why do you fear them?

   ....

5. Did you ever face these emotions in others before? If so, what happened?

....

Why You Fear Emotions

As you can probably see from your answers above, we tend to fear certain emotions, in ourselves and others, because they make us feel small, powerless, overwhelmed. This is caused by three main issues:

Adultism. We've all been small and we have probably all been shouted at, ridiculed, frightened by someone bigger than us. This might be a parent, carer, relative, brother or sister, school friend, passer-by, teacher, religious leader, and so on. When young people are hurt (through physical and verbal means) by someone older, it is called 'adultism'. When asked, most people can usually remember a punitive teacher, school bullies or unjust treatment from parents. Adultism is central to why we fear certain emotions, because they can remind us of the past when we were powerless and overwhelmed. (See also Chapter 3: Facing Where Addictions Begin, and Chapter 4: Facing Social Pressures.)

Mental Health System. Another brake on facing feelings is the 'bogey man' of the mental health system looming over us. We fear 'going mad', 'cracking up', 'breaking down'. The threat of being detained in a mental hospital is a major barrier against healthy emotional release. Many of my clients say they fear 'losing control' and ending up on tranquillizers, anti-depressants, sleeping pills or, worse, in a mental institution.

When you give up addictions, it is like pulling the cork out of the emotional bottle. You (and your nearest and dearest) can get very scared about what is going to come flying out. Although it is neither appropriate nor desirable that you go around 'dumping' your raw feelings on people, it is none the less necessary to be able to face your feelings in order to get off the hook. (See also Chapter 8: Making the Break, Chapter 9:

Being Your Own Parent, Chapter 10: Meeting Your Emotional Needs, and Chapter 17: Staying Free.)

Oppression. Not everybody is treated equally in our society, although they should be. For example, if you are female, young, black, disabled, elderly, non-English speaking, and/or working-class, you will probably be experiencing oppression (in some form or other) daily. Being treated less fairly is very painful, even if you think you have got used to it (and especially if you deny it exists).

People from disadvantaged groups often go to great lengths to look 'cool', believing that to reveal real unhappiness, anger, pain or fear would give away even more power to the oppressive society. So sub-cultures can be based on the suppression of overt emotions through using addictions. Even within disadvantaged groups, members can feel it is hard to show real feelings to each other. This can lead to conflict being turned inwards self-destructively, thereby weakening the group. Addictions also bind members together with a common cultural experience against a common foe. (See Chapter 7: Facing Oppression.)

HOW EMOTIONS WORK

As we have already seen, we have emotions for a reason: they are a natural mechanism for healing emotional and physical hurts. This is how they work.

If you get hurt emotionally, physically or both, and are unable to release (or completely release) feelings such as grief, fear, anger, surrounding the experience, a 'distress pattern' is created. Everything that occurs at the time of a distress experience is recorded: sights, sounds, smells, physical sensations, your emotional state at the time, the weather, and so on.

If hurtful experiences remain unreleased, they can accumulate into 'chronic distress'. This is a distress pattern which has become deeply ingrained by being reinforced over and over and over again. It is like a large 'snowball' of unreleased pain rolling downhill, gathering debris as it goes. Accumulated distress can become so compacted that it becomes impossible to separate the 'real' you from the chronic distress. When we talk about someone's 'personality', we are usually describing their chronic distress. When we say 'Darren's always miserable', or 'Anne's always so loud', or 'Peter worries all the time', we are actually pointing to their unreleased chronic distress.

Real Needs

Of course, we all have real needs that are very much related to our present-day lives. Here are the main ones. No doubt you could add others.

- Attention
- Love
- Affection
- Nourishment (food and drink when we need it)
- Safety
- Shelter
- Validation
- Communication
- Connection
- Mental stimulation
- Creativity
- Exercise
- Physical closeness

Because these needs are not always met adequately, especially during our early lives when we cannot articulate what we want, most of us grow up still feeling we need them to be met. (See also Chapter 3: Facing Where Addictions Begin.) In such circumstances those unfulfilled needs become frozen and much of our lives can be spent futilely trying to meet these needs.

Frozen Needs

These are real needs which were not met adequately (or at all) when we needed them to be met. For instance, if you were left alone to cry as a baby, your real needs at the time, for physical affection, love, security and perhaps for food, drink, and comfort, were not met. If you don't ever release the emotional pain around this kind of experience, a distress pattern can be established. In this case it would say, 'No-one is ever there when I need them, no matter how hard I cry'; or 'I'm not important, nobody loves me'; or 'I'm alone in the world, I have to do everything for myself – I can't trust anyone'.

This is how feelings of isolation and disconnection become established. If this experience is repeated over and over during childhood, the likelihood is you will grow up with a chronic distress recording, and find it difficult, if not impossible, to trust people with your deepest feelings. You can even feel this isolated while being a success both socially and at work, be married, have children, be surrounded by colleagues and family.

Being Listened To

We all have a real need to be listened to, but few of us ever are. One exercise I do at workshops is to get people into pairs and ask them to listen to each other, in turn, for five minutes. They are not to nod, ask questions, join in, comment, interrupt. People who are listened to usually feel that five minutes is like an hour. They feel under an uncomfortable spotlight and wriggle and giggle with embarrassment. They report wanting their partner to 'say something', and that the silence is unbearable. Others drink up the attention and pour out all sorts of worries and griefs. Meanwhile, the listener can feel very uncomfortable, not nodding or 'umming' with agreement. It can be very hard *not* to comment or interrupt, especially not to chip in with 'Yes, that's exactly how I feel', and pull the conversation's focus on to themselves.

We are all hungry for attention and thirsty for a good ear. Going out with friends is often an opportunity for having a good moan. However, these 'sessions' are more complicated than going to a professional counsellor, as you have to take care of the relationship (and network of relationships). Distress patterns become chronic because nobody listened at the time you needed to be listened to – and still nobody's listening, really listening, to what you need to say. If you have ever experienced a crisis, such as a death, a car accident or breaking a bone, you will probably have wanted to talk about it over and over to 'get it out of your system'. That is why the Samaritans are so immensely popular in the UK. They offer a dispassionate ear 24 hours a day, without judgement, comment or advice. Something we all need desperately and something which is entirely healthy and necessary to overcome our addictions.

Distress Patterns, Unmet Needs and Addictions

So what has any of this got to do with addictions? Quite simply, our addictions stem from our unreleased chronic distress patterns; in particular, from our frozen needs.

When Jean was seven her father died suddenly of a heart attack (she is now 56). She remembers the moment when she was told the news: 'A policeman knocked on the door and my mother was taken away suddenly. Then my sister told me we had to go to my aunt's nearby. I didn't understand what was going on and I was taken out into my aunt's garden, sat on a stool and asked if I knew where people went when they died. Being a good Christian little girl I said "Yes", and my sister and I chorused, "Heaven". Then my aunt said, "Well, your daddy has gone to Heaven with the angels," whereupon my sister and I began to cry. But I was told to stop because I was upsetting my sister.'

The two girls were then 'bribed' by their uncle not to show their feelings. 'We were told that if we stopped crying and behaved ourselves we'd be taken to the park. I was frightened of my uncle, so I stopped crying. My uncle also told me we had to be "brave", look after my mother and not make a fuss. My mother was the only one who was allowed to show any emotion – and that was snuffling into a hankie in a silent, embarrassed way. After that I didn't cry again until I was about 50.'

Jean had real needs as a child to be listened to and loved, so she could release her natural grief and fear at her father's death. Instead, she was shut up and made to feel other people's needs were more important. Shortly after this, Jean stopped eating and lost weight, and has continued to be anorexic ever since, her self-starvation getting worse at times of emotional stress. By 20, Jean was a heavy smoker and drinker and on anti-depressants. She ended up in mental hospital and only in her fifties is she finally realizing that having and showing feelings is entirely appropriate and natural.

Her 'frozen needs' for attention, affection and love have led her to have disastrous relationships where she's been the one to give too much and live a 'tragically lonely' life. In other words, she is constantly re-enacting that hurtful experience as a seven-year-old, in the vain hope that someone will finally come and make her feel better.

In my experience there is always a direct link between unreleased distress, frozen needs and addiction. It is the driving force behind 'The Addictive Treadmill'. We are hungry, needy, empty, thirsty, and we feel hollow inside. We want to feel full, satisfied, satiated, quenched. The stark truth is frozen needs can never be filled, no matter how hard you try. It is an illusion to believe you can. The desire to fill frozen needs can be irresistible, even drive you to crimes of passion or desperate risk-taking. Whether it is the urge to make a million, eat vats of ice-cream or have wild love affairs, the engine of desire behind the addiction is the same – chronic distress and frozen needs.

In order to give up your addictions you have to acknowledge that forceful desires derive from where you feel insatiably needy (metaphorically hungry and thirsty), hurt, unloved and ignored. Only then can emotional healing occur.

EMOTIONAL HEALING

We are all born with an innate mechanism for emotional healing. If not interfered with, you will feel and release your feelings quite naturally. For instance.

- When you feel sad, lose someone/something or are physically hurt, you will cry.

- When you feel frustrated, you will get angry, irritable, even rage.

- When you're frightened, you will shake, sweat, and/or scream.

- When you're embarrassed or shy, you will laugh (a form of light fear).

- When you're recovering from physical tensions, hurts, anaesthetics and/or drugs (including the use of chemical addictions), you will yawn. Yawning isn't just getting more air, being bored or wanting to go to sleep; it has a profound healing purpose.

Unfortunately, most of us have had this natural means of emotional healing interfered with, so healing doesn't take place easily. This means we can go through life with a lot of unnecessary pain, which limits functioning, distorts our perceptions and makes it hard to trust, love, care, grow, take risks, fulfil our potential.

Our culture has lots of taboos about showing feelings, which causes additional hurts to be implanted through ridicule, punishment and social sanctions, as we saw in Jean's case above. It is still thought to be rude, vulgar and excessive to release many emotions publicly. Even in private, people can grow up with their emotions tightly repressed. Over the past 20 years it has become more acceptable for men to cry more openly and for women to be angry. However, we still have a long way to go. (See also Chapter 3: Facing Social Pressures.)

Breakdown or Break-through?

Most people are terrified of 'breaking down' when their emotions rise to the surface uncontrollably. And, indeed, if you experience a crisis, such as a relationship ending, the death of a child or losing a job, your emotions can feel overwhelming. Few of us have escaped feeling depressed, frightened, grief-stricken, when it seems too much bother to get up, go out or even eat. The hardest thing to do in these circumstances is to reach out and ask for help. Yet that is precisely what has to be done, to combat the fear and isolation that overwhelming emotions can evoke.

I always tell clients that they are having a 'break-through' rather than a breakdown. The spectre of mental illness keeps too many people silent in their suffering. It is much more healthy to recognize, even welcome, strong emotions, even if at the time it feels as if they're going to engulf you. Inevitably, times of crisis and depression are part of the process of emotional healing. Perhaps in mid-life you fall ill or divorce, and out tumbles all the old, unresolved pain of your earlier life. Perhaps you hit the bottle, perhaps you turn to drugs, or compulsive sex, to numb out the pain. Ironically, although these times are gruelling, they can be periods of enormous personal growth, the rewards of which can be reaped for the rest of your life. Deciding to stay with the pain, and release it systematically without numbing yourself out with chemical and emotional addictions, can change your life, and be a positive break-through, instead of a negative breakdown.

Even if you end up taking tranquillizers, anti-depressants or sleeping pills for a short period due to the enormity of your emotional pain, all is not lost. Sometimes these drugs can be helpful (although ideally undesirable) as a temporary bridge between a terrifying event and recovery. If short-lived, medically supervised with a view to coming off as soon as possible, these sorts of drugs can have a limited use. However, they are *never* a short-cut to the process of emotional healing that needs to occur naturally to aid recovery. Always insist on having drugs which will still enable you to grieve and function (this means avoiding drugs like Valium, Librium and Largactil which numb your senses, hindering the natural healing process). As soon as you can, you need to come off any interim medication, having built the support and received the medical advice you need to do so. Never, ever, stop these kinds of drugs without proper, qualified supervision – it can be very dangerous.

'Reminders'

We probably spend 99 per cent of the time with our attention on past hurts instead of living fully in the present. Whether we know it or not, we are constantly searching for a way to release past pain so we can heal ourselves emotionally. 'Reminders' trigger the proverbial majority of the emotional iceberg hidden under the water level. For instance, a romantic or tragic love-story may remind you of unreleased pain from early separations, losses, abandonments, broken friendships, sibling deaths, as well as current relationship breakdowns.

Reminders will always abound, precisely because film-makers, writers, and dramatists reflect and analyse the human condition constantly. If you don't want to be a victim of reminders, you can make a decision ahead of time that you will not be 'set off' by what you see and/or you will avoid being reminded. We use memorabilia like films, songs, scents such as perfume or after-shave, family photo-albums, often completely unawarely, to evoke unreleased emotions in an instant because we are always hoping to heal.

The Benefits of Emotional Healing

- You can live in the present and not be sunk in the past or anxious about the future.

- You feel more relaxed, sleep better, feel more centred.

- You don't fear feelings. You harness their energy for your own good.

- You don't fear other people's feelings. You accept, even welcome, their displays of emotion as part of their humanness.

- You learn to recognize feelings and plan for their release. So, take a good friend and some tissues to a weepy movie, and enjoy. Don't stifle back valuable tears any longer. It is a waste of a good healing session.

- Physical health improves, because you are in balance. Stifled emotions nearly always come out in physical symptoms, such as migraines, irritable bowel syndrome, influenza, and in extreme cases of severe emotional repression, with chronic illnesses like ME (Myalgic-encephalomyelitis) and life-threatening diseases such as cancer.

- You feel powerful and really more in control – because nothing can surprise you (you're no longer at the mercy of your own unbridled feelings). You accept yourself more, and never again need to apologize for 'making a fuss' or 'breaking down'. You can learn to celebrate and welcome your emotionality instead.

- You come alive – to smells, tastes, beauty, colours, love, music, people, fun, exciting experiences, nature, happiness – because you have thawed out layers of fear, sadness, mistrust and anger.

In Chapter 8: Making the Break, and Chapter 9: Being Your Own Parent, I will explain how to identify your own frozen and real needs; and in Chapter 10: Meeting Your Emotional Needs, I describe the practicalities of handling your emotions in order to get off the hook. But first of all it is essential to understand where your own addictions began.

Chapter 3

———— o ————

Facing Where Addictions Begin

Do you know your early life story? Stressful experiences from the beginning of your life until now have shaped the nature and extent of your chemical and emotional addictions — especially if the emotional pain surrounding these experiences has not been released successfully. This chapter will explain how your experience of pre-birth, birth, childhood, family/parents, school, student and work life helped you get hooked.

PRE-BIRTH EXPERIENCES

From the moment your father's sperm penetrated your mother's ovum, you were alive and beginning to grow. Yet, a developing foetus is still often (wrongly) thought of as an unfeeling lump. Unlike in China, where the months spent in the womb are counted towards a child's age, our own culture discounts the first nine months of life, so that we only start counting our lives from the first day of birth. Yet, the growing foetus is capable of perceiving and processing complex information through the placenta and its own cells. Later in pregnancy, the baby's own sensory equipment can experience sound, light, movement, and emotional and physical changes in both itself and in its mother. It is therefore logical to assume that an unborn baby can also experience distress, whether due to its mother's physical and/or emotional states, or due to its own independent experiences.

Today, we are increasingly aware of the importance of pre-natal care. Pregnant women are generally more conscious of the need to give up harmful habits, such as smoking cigarettes (and passive smoking by inhaling other people's cigarette smoke), as well as the dangers of alcohol, junk food, illegal drugs, antibiotics, caffeine, painkillers, and so on. Where there is little knowledge and/or care taken during pregnancy, a baby can be born underweight and/or premature, possibly disabled and with addictions to substances such as nicotine, alcohol and crack. I know something about this from my own pre-natal experience.

My Own Pre-birth and Early Life

My own early life was fairly traumatic. My mother suffered from anaemia and general poor health, aggravated by grow-ing up during the Second World War. Blitz bombing and other terrifying experiences had left her extremely nervous and in poor health, and I was conceived while rationing was still a part of everyday life during the early fifties. Little was understood then about the effects of poor diet, smoking cigarettes, drinking alcohol, prescribed drugs, the emotional state of parents and environmental factors on a foetus. I think I consumed quite a few drugs and experienced a lot of fear while growing in my mother's womb.

I *was* a wanted baby. In fact, there were two of us – I had a male twin who was tragically miscarried late in the pregnancy. Like my mother, I also had a rare rhesus blood group and my birth was long and exhausting; we both nearly died. I was born prematurely, with a club-foot (which, fortunately, was straightened during my first year of life by Great Ormond Street Hospital, in London). I also spent the first months of my babyhood in an incubator and was not breastfed.

My parents never told me about my club foot, believing it was a shameful secret that should remain hidden (there were no full-length photos of me as a baby). I only uncovered the story of my twin and my disability through counselling in my twenties, where I also got in touch with very early feelings of terror, loss, rejection and isolation. Very often I would automatically curl into a foetus-shaped ball during a counselling session, with arms and legs crossed and fists clenched and shake and cry while being reassured and held by my counsellor. I didn't believe I was really 'remembering' at first, but the sensations were powerful and I now know that losing my brother and being in the incubator was extremely traumatic for me. I felt abandoned, isolated and punished for being born disabled. I have 'remembered' the adults around me expressing a lot of anxiety, disappointment and even disgust about my disability. I did not thrive at first and had a long, lonely struggle to stay alive. When, in my twenties, I finally told my mother about my revelations she burst into tears, amazed that I could have uncovered the whole story as she had never spoken to me (or anyone else) about it.

I am very glad I made it through, because I love being alive, but I believe my later addictions developed from these early experiences. I have been looking (fruitlessly) for my lost twin all my life: I have had a string of intense best-friendships and passionate soul-mate relationships, with a constant longing to be 'joined at the hip' with someone. This has led me to be emotionally addicted to love and sex as a means of getting close physical contact, and I have also been a compulsive carer-codependent. I have always felt deeply guilty because I survived at my twin's expense.

My difficulty in thriving also developed into anorexia and drink-related addictions in my teens and twenties (not only alcohol, but endless hot drinks, especially tea). I always starved myself when upset and feared not getting enough to drink, especially during the night, and I am still a very oral person. I love being in water – baths, swimming pools, jacuzzis – in fact, anything womb-like, warm, watery, and safe. I need masses of hugs and physical contact – so when I feel isolated, this is precisely what gets me back to planet earth. I have howled many hundreds of hours, hanging limpet-close on to trusted, loving counsellors, grieving the loss of my twin, the lack of bonding with my mother and my isolation through being 'exiled' in a glass box.

Clients' Pre-birth Experiences

Because of my awareness about the importance of pre-birth life I have been able to help many people uncover the root of their own addictions in order to get off the hook. Knowledge is power and feeling powerful is a key contradiction to feeling a small, vulnerable, dependent victim. However, you may find the concept of pre-birth life unbelievable, frightening, even laughable. Some clients have found it easier to believe in having a 'past-life' as a Roman soldier than the reality of facing their first nine months in the womb. With counselling, we have usually discovered that their resistance is due to needing to deny the truth of painful events occurring while they were developing. I might ask 'What's your earliest memory connected with your mother?' or 'What's your earliest memory connected to being in the womb?' and then encourage the client to trust their 'first thought'. Often clients feel they can't speak, and just roll up small, shake and cry, feeling very vulnerable and bewildered.

John, a 24-year-old sales representative, who came to an addictions workshop to try to give up drugs, got very angry when I asked him what happened while he was in his mother's womb. He was clearly frightened and instantly attacked me verbally, almost physically. We later stayed with this feeling over several sessions and eventually uncovered memories of his father beating up his mother late in pregnancy. Indeed, this young man knew his father was a violent drunk during his childhood and teens, but it was too terrifying for him to accept that similar abuse had occurred when he was tiny. When he did finally understand and accept the truth, and started releasing his fear, grief and outrage, his emotional healing accelerated. He was able to stop abusing himself through the violence of drugs, compulsive TV-watching (especially violent films), and compulsive love, sex, over-eating, fitness training and reckless driving.

Other clients have uncovered frightening pre-birth memories about near-miscarriages, attempted abortions, parental sexual intercourse as well as *pleasant* memories of music, travel and feelings of benign well-being and peace. This is clearly an area ripe for further research – which could well change the hopeless face of addiction as we know it. You may well find the idea of pre-birth life very disturbing, but there is a growing body of evidence from the work, observations and personal experiences of therapists, counsellors, perinatal researchers, healers, doctors, gynaecologists in the UK and abroad. In *Hidden Loss: Miscarriage and Ectopic Pregnancy*, (see 'Help' section), there is a fascinating account by Catherine Itzin about her own experience in the womb of near-miscarriage.

YOUR EARLY LIFE STORY

So what do you know about your own early life story? First of all, how do you feel about the question? What feelings does it bring up? Write down your 'first thoughts' in your note book.

....

....

You may know nothing, or very little, about your first nine months because, as a culture, we generally pay little attention to this time. Or you may have been told a few anecdotes about your mother eating eels and ice-cream at three in the morning. Try answering the following questions, again jotting down your 'first thoughts':

1. When and where were you conceived?

....

2. Were you planned or an 'accident'?

....

3. Were you wanted or not?

....

4. Was your gender wanted or not (i.e. did they want a girl or boy – were you welcomed for what you were?)

....

5. Were you an addition to a family? If so, were you the second, third, fourth child, etc?

....

6. Did your parent(s) ever consider or try an abortion? If so, what method was used?

....

7. Were you a near or threatened miscarriage?

....

8. Did you ever have a twin? If so, what happened?

....

9. Did other foetuses share your mother's womb with you? If 'Yes', how many?

....

10. Did your mother experience any accidents/serious illnesses while pregnant with you?

....

11. What were the external circumstances like – was there a war on, was there tension over money, housing, work, and so on? Was there an election or national calamity? Were there other children around in your home already?

....

12. What was the weather like during the pregnancy, especially during the latter stages?

....

13. What was the state of mind of your parent(s) during the pregnancy?

....

14. How was your own health during your mother's pregnancy?

....

15. Did your mother have an amniocentesis test (to see if you were disabled)?

....

16. Were you born with any kind of disability (no matter how trivial)? If so, what happened?

....

17. Did your mother smoke, drink alcohol, take legal or illegal drugs during your pregnancy?

....

18. How was her diet? Did she have any eating disorders?

....

19. How was your birth? How long did it take? What kind of delivery was it? Were drugs involved? Were you hospitalized in any way? Was it at home, in hospital, in a taxi? Were there 'complications'?

....

20. Were you breastfed? fed to the clock? or on demand? Did you sleep in or by your mother's bed or were you separated? Were you in an incubator?

....

21. Who was around in the first few days, weeks and months of your life? Was it a calm, loving atmosphere? Or was it stressful? Was there poverty or plenty, or what?

....

22. Were you adopted? If so, do you know what happened to you directly after your birth and during the first few months?

....

Look at your notebook answers – what do they tell you about you? How did you feel about doing this quiz? Did it seem relevant or irrelevant? Did you feel angry? Fascinated? Upset to realize you knew so little? Bored? Pleased your early life was so good? Confused – can't remember a thing? Write down your 'first thoughts' in your notebook.

....

Look back at your notes for Chapter 1, where you identified your addictions. Do you see any links between your early life story with any current eating, drinking, spending habits, etc.?

....

Are there any clues you can follow to understand yourself more? (If you are in contact with your parent(s) or family at large, you may want to use these questions to find out more.)

....

As we saw in Chapter 2, addictions largely come from unreleased chronic distress, especially your isolation and frozen needs. So the more information you have the better you should be able to understand *why* you have developed your own particular addictions.

PARENTS: HANDLING EMOTIONS

Being a parent is a tough job, particularly nowadays when young couples may live far away from their own parents and be largely thrown on their own resources. There's no training, little support and nearly everyone is worried about getting it wrong. The growing of the next generation is an essential, labour-intensive task which most parents struggle to learn on

the job. One of the toughest challenges of parenting is learning to handle your own and your children's emotions. The
reason so many parents (and other adults) have so much
discomfort around their children's emotional release is because of the pressure of their own bottled up emotions. (See
Chapter 2.)

We all know new-born babies make a lot of noise. Yet very
few of us encourage them to give full reign to their feelings
because of particular prejudices about the natural process of
emotional healing which occurs with emotional release. So
encouraging children to let rip is often seen as:

- A sign of weakness ('big boys don't cry, don't be a cry-baby').

- An unpleasant reminder to parents and carers of their own
  early hurts and emotions (which they were probably stopped from expressing fully or at all). Some babies are still
  silenced by dummies and other 'comforters' (including
  alcohol, food and sugar). They are also controlled by
  punishments such as being left to cry alone and/or being
  shouted at, hit or threatened.

- A symptom of being a bad, undisciplined parent (that is, a
  'good' baby is a quiet baby and any screaming, crying,
  raging, is a sign of a baby being 'bad', undisciplined and/or
  badly brought up).

- Wilfulness on the part of the baby, trying to manipulate
  busy and exhausted parents into 'spoiling' him or her with
  too much attention.

- A sign of the devil (or similar evil force).

These ideas are clearly based on misinformation. The fact that
they are popular doesn't mean they are right. Babies express
their feelings for a reason, and it is not always just to do with
dirty nappies and a need for food. A new-born infant has had
a plethora of emotional experiences during the nine-month
gestation period. And this is followed by the exhausting and
frightening experience of being born – leaving the darkness
and security of the womb for the bright lights and challenges
of a hospital delivery room, or bedroom. Babies have to adjust

to a strange, noisy environment and a new regime of wearing clothes, learning to feed, sleeping in light and dark places, being alone, being held, talked to, physically handled by nurses, doctors, parents, and so on. If a baby needs special medical attention and is separated from his or her mother for long periods during this initial bonding stage, this can install feelings of powerlessness and isolation.

Fortunately, today, premature and sickly babies are touched, hugged, talked to, and kept in close contact with their mothers as much as possible, to combat isolation. How a baby learns to feed, whether breast-fed or not, and whether he or she is fed on demand or to a timetable will influence eating patterns in later life.

Parents' Own Emotions

Some parents feel hugely anxious when their offspring cry, others feel almost irrepressible anger and impatience. Few are relaxed and take it completely in their stride. Parents' emotional responses to their baby's crying, and other expressions of emotion, provide a direct route to their own early experiences. Were new parents given caring attention when their own tensions were triggered off by their children's emotional outbursts, they would probably surprise themselves by producing rivers of unreleased tears and torrents of repressed rage.

Janet, a 32-year-old schoolteacher, told me about her uncontrollable urge to punish her baby and smash his head against the wall when he screamed, especially at night. 'I would have this uncontrollable feeling of being about to snap and had to go out of the room or bash something, sometimes my own fist on the wall, to stop me doing it. It really scared me, because I felt I would crack any minute.' Janet had no idea before she had a baby that she would find this screaming quite so stressful. She thought it would be hard, but not as incredibly difficult as she found it. She phoned Cry-sis, the organization which offers 24-hour telephone advice for parents unable to cope with their crying babies, when desperate at 4 am and when she was 'on the edge of bashing him'. With counselling help she began to uncover her own experiences as a baby, being repeatedly chastised by her angry father. As she grieved, shook and raged, the urge to hurt her child diminished and she was eventually able to listen to his screams with a degree of equanimity.

Because counselling help is not widely available, most parents have to cope the best they can, reinforcing what they believe are the 'good' and 'bad' emotions in their children (See Chapter 2). Rewards, in the shape of food, cuddles, praise ('good boy'), are given when children are quiet and docile. Punishment, by withdrawal of love and approval, or infliction of verbal violence: 'naughty girl', and/or smacks, can be doled out for crying, screaming, raging and other forms of emotional release.

The Problem of Gender Stereotyping

How parents treat boys and girls from birth is clearly important for the development of their gender identity. A brave vanguard of parents is throwing away the pink and blue bootees along with the toy guns and Barbie dolls. But most parents report that it is very hard to scotch stereotyping, especially once children go to play- and primary school.

Despite 30 years of Women's Liberation (and now Men's Liberation), boys and girls, men and women are still treated differently. We expect boys to be tougher, less emotional, brave and active, angry, but not soppy. Girls are still expected to be soft, caring, more emotional and passive. We expect women to weep, but not to rage. Although the social climate is slowly changing, it can still be hard for men to express their emotions as openly as women, and for both genders to express the whole spectrum of emotions. Clearly, if parents become more comfortable with the expression of *all* emotions, regardless of gender, their offspring will be able to do the same. Getting practical support would help parents to do this.

FAMILY AND HOME: WHAT'S NORMAL?

Families can take many forms: single parent, separated and divorced, living together, extended (with aunts, grandparents, in-laws), lesbian or gay, communal as well as the traditional unit of mum, dad and 1.7 children. Children learn many things from their parents, including addictive behaviours. You tend to think what your family does is 'normal' – but what is normal?

'I don't remember a great deal about my childhood,' explains Hazel, a 42-year-old administrator and single parent, 'but I do remember I once got everyone drunk by about ten o'clock at a family party. I was eight and my job was to go round pouring drinks. My father got very cross with me, but I said "Daddy, I'm just pouring out the same drinks as I do for you". What I didn't know then was that he was an alcoholic.' Hazel's mother was hooked on tranquillizers and equally 'not there' emotionally. 'It sounds absurd, but I used to go and look through other people's windows to see what "normal" family life was like. I longed for something just like on the Oxo-adverts.' Real life is clearly a lot more messy than the advertisements on TV would have us believe.

Unhappy Families

If a family is unhappy, through chemical and emotional addictions, relationship breakdown, or other problems, but nothing is done about it, children can grow up damaged. It can seem as if there is a pink elephant sitting in the middle of the room. Instead of acknowledging it is there, the adults squeeze past it or pretend it is not there at all. This can leave children feeling very confused about reality. Is mum or dad drunk, stoned, angry or what? Are they really just tired? Children often feel they're to blame for their parents' weird behaviour, and the fear and self-loathing this confusion creates can lead to addictions in later life.

Smart, middle-class Samantha, aged 35, seems flawless. Yet, when she talks about her childhood, she suddenly looks tragic. 'Mealtimes were terrible. I spent my time being the peace-maker. I wanted to keep up the pretence that everything was all right, although we all knew, somehow, that it was not. I spent a lot of time anticipating what people were going to do or say, and trying to work out how everyone else was feeling. If my mother, who was a drinker, snapped at my brother, I would intervene and deflect the dart. If my father, who was a workaholic, was absent through being still at work, I would distract everybody with funny stories. It was a terrible effort and inside I was screaming "why can't we just talk about what's going on?"'

The family never did talk about their 'pink elephant' and Samantha only got to break the silence when she underwent treatment for her own bulimia. 'The pretence that everything was fine while it clearly wasn't drove me mad, so I pretended to eat normally while bingeing and throwing up in secret. My bulimia was like a mirror-image of our whole family. I felt so awful I was hell bent on destroying my own body by self-abuse. Then maybe *someone* would do *something*.'

Self-Esteem

Families are crucial in building, or demolishing, your self-esteem. Let's suppose babies are benign, intelligent beings when born who need to be welcomed, respected and loved. So, how you are treated from birth will clearly impact upon how you grow up. Obviously, if you are told that you are bad, naughty, wicked, and are hit, threatened, ignored, beaten, ridiculed, sexually abused, neglected, teased, punished, laughed at, scapegoated, blamed, your self-esteem will be extremely low. While if you are told (and shown) that you're good, deserving, lovable, intelligent, worthwhile, respected, physically attractive, talented, bright, and that you have rights, then your self-esteem will be high.

'Spoiling'

We are often more worried about 'spoiling' children than concerned about them developing a positive sense of self-worth. Of course, spoiling doesn't arise from telling someone they are good and lovable, or giving them attention when they need it, it comes from misguided permissiveness. Children need firm frameworks, you have to say 'no' and set limits, but this can be done with love, respect, understanding and care for the inevitable emotional reaction. It is important to hold a child close or 'be there' for them, and give loving attention while they rage, cry, and struggle out their anger and grief. They will stop quite naturally sooner or later and their attention will move on to something new and interesting. The problem for parents in this situation is that their own feelings can get in the way of staying with the child's emotional release. A child is only 'spoilt' if parents, fearing the emotional reaction, appease and confuse by 'giving in' inappropriately, when tantrums are thrown to gain points.

Sharing

Sharing is important in family life. Sometimes there is inequality, such as when the boys and men get the best food, or the girls and women get the most comfortable beds. Or there's intense rivalry between father and son, mother and daughter, or between siblings. Learning to share is an important part of growing up and some people feel bitter that they have not had their fair share. Usually this is to do with their real needs (for food, drink, affection, love, validation, attention) not having been met, so their frozen needs become a driving force. If you find it hard to share, you probably feel resentful about not having had enough. You might be greedy and/or a compulsive eater. You can feel starved both physically and emotionally and develop cunning, secretive, anti-social and addictive patterns of behaviour as a consequence. You may not be conscious that you are doing this – but you'll probably experience a lot of anxiety about not getting enough when out for a meal with friends or be envious of other people's successes and acquisitions. Your addiction may not even be attached to the same thing you missed out on first time around, but the distress pattern will be there if it has not had a chance to be worked on.

Treats

'Treats' are usually the 'punishment and reward' system in family life. Treats are usually things such as chocolate, fizzy drinks, sweets, ice-cream, but can also be privileges: extra pocket money, watching TV and/or staying up late. Treats are a bargaining tool, whereby parents buy themselves peace and obedience. However, treats can backfire:

- By making sweet things 'special', and 'wholesome' foods boring.

- By enabling parents to manipulate their children's behaviour, which can in turn teach their children to manipulate others.

- By making life a series of goals to be met with 'treats' with little ongoing enjoyment in between.

'I'm a compulsive cake eater,' confesses 65-year-old Bryony. 'I was brought up very strictly. Sugary things were a special treat. I had to be especially good, like having passed my exams well, to have some.' Bryony finds herself unable to go past a cake shop without going in and buying at least five different cakes. Her compulsive eating started in earnest when she was under pressure as a young mother, feeling very alone with a screaming toddler. 'Cakes were treats. David could have food when he wanted, so why couldn't I? I ended up cleaning up his plate and shoving all the left-overs in my mouth as fast as possible. I didn't want anyone to see. I'm still very secretive about it and feel very embarrassed about owning up. But I notice that when I feel lonely and unhappy I still find myself craving. I feel life is hard enough without me having to resist, but I hardly ever stop at one because I feel I deserve more. I feel good while I'm doing it, but bad immediately after for having done it – then I'm filled with remorse and self-loathing.'

Bryony knows she is hooked on the sugar as a chemical addiction, and the food as a 'treat'. The problem is cakes can't solve her feelings of loneliness. Bryony is on the Addictive Treadmill described in Chapter 2, with a sugar 'high', followed by 'come down' sugar blues, which requires another sugar 'high', and so on. (See also *Sugar Blues* by William Dufty listed in the 'Help' section.)

Boredom and Isolation

We can all remember moments of intense boredom in childhood. Perhaps it was sitting still with the 'grown ups', or being indoors when it was raining, or being exiled to your room in punishment, being in hospital or in bed ill. If you are bored, you are usually under-stimulated mentally, need attention and connection with others. That means you are isolated as well. Only and eldest children can get very bored because they're either often alone or overloaded with responsibility. Resorting to chemical and/or emotional addictions can be a way of coping with the pain of boredom.

Alice and her brother Mark were staying with an aunt while their parents were on holiday. Alice was 10, her brother eight. 'Auntie spent all her time in the kitchen and we were missing mum and dad, so one afternoon we locked ourselves in the living room and slugged our way through the booze cupboard. We both went green and threw up, but it beat the boredom all right,' remembers Alice, now 37. Fear of being bored can motivate a lot of adults to keep numb by using chemical and emotional addictions. Long-term, it is better to cure the boredom (and/or release the old feelings) than resort to self-abuse through addiction.

Sexual Abuse, Physical Abuse and Neglect

Some families harbour sexual abuse, physical abuse and neglect of children. This kind of mistreatment cuts across class, race and culture: its extent is far greater than most of us realize, or want to acknowledge. But what has it got to do with addiction?

Addictive substances are often used to tempt children to do things they instinctively know are wrong. The man in the mac who uses sweets to bribe children into allowing sexual abuse (and silence about that abuse) is actually out there. And it's not just strangers who commit such abuse; it's fathers, mothers, sisters, brothers, uncles, grandfathers, and babysitters, too.

'When I was 10, my dad used to say, "come upstairs, I've got something for you",' remembers Bea, now 22. 'I was then told I'd get double my pocket money if I did what he wanted. I'd have to go down on all fours and pretend I was sweeping the floor while he pulled up my skirt and had anal sex with me. It hurt like hell and I was very frightened because my dad was very strong. He would then put jam on his penis and make me lick it off. Afterwards he'd give me the money and a slice of bread and jam, the same jam, and make me eat it in front of him. I used to gag, and to this day I can't eat cheap raspberry jam, it makes me utterly sick.' Bea is now self-employed as a cleaner and a prostitute.

Sexual and physical abuse are violations of children's basic rights. At the moment of the abuse the child is no longer safe, respected or loved. The child's real needs for safety, love, affection and attention are not met. If these hurts are not released, then they can become chronic distress which says:

- 'I'm not lovable.'

- 'I'm deeply bad.'

- 'There's something wrong with me.'

- 'I have to earn love by letting people do what they want with me.'

- 'Sex/love/caring is always exchanged for money, treats and/or goods.'

Neglect makes a child feel worthless and undeserving of good treatment. This can destroy a child's self-esteem and result in patterns of self-punishment and abuse. Such children usually have a mass of frozen needs, which can lead to addiction.

Do As I Do, Not As I Say

If parents' addictive behaviour is evident in the home, children will probably copy it. In *Growing Up In Smoke* (See 'Help' section), Lynne Michell's survey results showed that children raised in smoking environments tended to end up smokers. This is true of Barry, now 50. 'I have fond childhood memories of seeing my pregnant mother relaxing with her feet up, a cigarette in one hand and coffee mug balanced on her belly. All my life I've associated a cup of coffee and a cigarette with relaxation. I still smoke 40 a day, and drink masses of coffee, as a consequence. I really have no idea how I'd relax any other way.'

While Barry is nostalgic about his mother's addictions, some young people – 16-year-old Dawn, from Edinburgh, for example – are frightened by them. 'I always hated my mum smoking. We'd had lessons about smoking at primary school, I had read about it in magazines and had seen programmes on TV. I was frightened that she would die from lung cancer. I also hated breathing in the smoke and my hair and clothes smelt awful.' Dawn helped her mother give up smoking but, more important, feels that her mother has earned the right to tell her not to smoke. 'Before, when she told me the dangers of smoking, I'd say, "How can you say that when you still do it, mum?"' In fact, Dawn copied her mum with the odd puff behind the school shed. 'I didn't like it. I respect mum more because she's now doing what she tells me to do.' Clearly, expecting your children to do what you do, rather than just what you say, has greater impact.

There are many clues to your chemical and emotional addictions buried in your early and family life. What rang bells for you in this chapter? Note down your responses in your notebook, as before.

1. Did your parents have addictions? What were they and how did you feel about it? Do you see any links between your addictions and theirs?

....

2. How did you feel about sharing? Were you bored? Isolated?

....

3. Were you ever abused, sexually or physically, or neglected? Can you see any links with your own addictions?

....

4. Did you have treats? If so, what? What role do treats play in your life now?

....

THE FULL PICTURE

This chapter has necessarily looked at the bleaker sides of early and family life. This doesn't mean to say that you did not have fun on holiday, at weekends, at home, or that everything was unrelentingly bad. You may well have good memories about times in your family when people 'let their hair down' and enjoyed themselves using addictions (can you remember times you all had fun without them?). Whatever the case for you, it's important to highlight that what you usually take for granted as 'normal' can create your addictions. You always need to keep in mind: 'Am I in control of my addictions, or do they control me?' As we have seen, addictions are rooted in everyday life – and especially in low self-esteem, feeling bored, blamed, isolated, unloved and/or abused, while being stopped from healing emotional pain. Central to getting off the hook is understanding more about why you are as you are, so you can be powerful about meeting your real needs for yourself.

Of course, we are also affected by our first independent social relationships and experiences at school, as students, trainees and at work. We'll explore these issues in the next chapter.

Chapter 4

———■◦■———

Facing Social Pressures

What do you do when you are under pressure? Have a nice cup of tea? Go out and get drunk? Slump in front of the TV with a 6-pack of beer? Eat several bars of chocolate? Disappear into a junk novel? Masturbate over pornography? Play video games? Play a hard game of squash? Attack the garden? Shout at the children? Phone a friend for hours and moan? Go out and spend money? Drive the car too fast? Daydream? Get yourself a new lover? Pick a fight or a row? Kick the cat?

COPING MECHANISMS

You have probably developed your own repertoire of coping mechanisms to deal with everyday social pressures. Some you will be fairly aware of – say, having a cup of coffee and a chocolate bar when you're exhausted. Others, such as masturbating over pornography, or picking up a new lover, you might keep secret, or be very ashamed of, not really acknowledging to yourself why or when you do it.

Addictions are our most favourite way of numbing out pressure – it has been said that there would be a social revolution overnight if we removed our everyday 'props' of sugar, caffeine, alcohol, nicotine and junk food/reading/videos and so on. We probably couldn't put up with impossible demands on time, energy, and health by working in goldfish-bowl offices, doing two full-time jobs as parent and employee, or put life and limb in danger doing hazardous hard-labour, because we would feel more of the pain, exhaustion, stress which gets blocked out by our addictions. Life is very pressurized and most of us keep going by running round and round on the 'Addictive Treadmill'. As you saw in Chapter 3, we have usually learned all sorts of bad habits from early life, most of which are founded on keeping the cork in the emotional bottle.

THE PRESSURES OF ADVERTISING

Advertising also plays a crucial role in getting us hooked. Advertisements shape our tastes, feed our fears and insecurities, remind us that we are vulnerable, needy and imperfect. They tease us that perfection is just out of reach, if only we stretched our pockets far enough to consume more of the right things.

Advertisements say:

- With their product you will feel better, look better, be liked more, be more successful, have better sex, more friends and the life you've always wanted.

- You need something artificial outside of yourself to succeed and 'feel good'.

- Eating sugar, chocolate, biscuits, cakes; drinking alcohol, tea, coffee, sweet fizzy drinks; smoking cigarettes and cigars; buying expensive cars, perfume, cosmetics, cameras; taking out more loans, insurance policies; having more expensive holidays – will solve all of your problems, and create none.

- Your fantasies are justifiable and stark reality would be palatable – if only you consumed more.

- Instant, 'harmless' pleasure is available effortlessly through opening a can, a tin, a bottle, a packet, or even a bank account.

Because advertising operates on a slick psychological level it invades our subconscious, making us want to reach out and buy without really having to think. We have learned from radio, TV, billboards, magazines that the perfect 'pick-me-up' is sitting on a supermarket shelf, ready to help us survive life's onslaughts. It is not that we don't know we are being manipulated; we do and we even enjoy it, as advertising has become almost a national art form and sport. The issue is really to face how much time, energy, artistic effort, money and resources go into selling us things which can even damage us ultimately. The main problem lies in our denial of the power of advertising to trigger our frozen needs, hungers and thirsts, thereby getting us well and truly hooked.

POLITICS AND ADDICTION

Governments and multi-national companies also play a large part in getting us addicted. Their position can seem very confusing because on the one hand, the Government is the guardian of public health and has a duty to promote a life free of addiction to smoking, drinking, eating too much of the wrong foods, getting into debt, driving too fast, etcetera, as both desirable and necessary. On the other hand, the Government (and the multi-nationals) reap huge financial benefits through revenues generated at home and abroad by selling addictive substances, such as tobacco and alcohol, and from interest accrued on credit card debts, and loans of all kinds.

The Government could only really be tough on addiction were they not to profit from it. And in a free-market economy, the Government does very little to curb multi-national production or advertising of addictive substances. Unfortunately, the price of addiction is high – it costs millions of lost work-hours, it costs the National Health Service (NHS) millions in health care for self-inflicted, avoidable disease, and it greatly reduces the quality of life. In the end we are the losers – we pay for the goods, we then also pay for healing ourselves from the effects of the goods (through the National Health Service and private health care/alternative therapies). This may seem a gloomy picture, but it is important to look outside of ourselves and face the social pressures that help us get hooked.

SCHOOL PRESSURES

School also generates social pressures which help us get addicted. Once you start going to a child minder or playschool, from a very early age you are being trained to be a social being. You will come under all sorts of pressures in having to fit into a group, learning to take your turn, being understimulated sometimes and overstretched and confused at others, dealing with competition, having to stand your ground in fights, being bullied by other children, being picked on by teachers. You may not feel you belong, maybe speaking one language at school and another at home, being with children from different backgrounds from your own, eating only at rigid mealtimes, having to produce work and have it evaluated in front of everyone, being organized and accountable.

School teachers and Heads are under constant pressure themselves and may have little time to give the emotional support that each child really needs. Sometimes children are struggling with very serious difficulties (from dyslexia to sexual abuse and back) and a caring, astute teacher will step in and help. But other children suffer in a private hell, unable to articulate either at school or at home what the problem is and instead sit on a mountain of unreleased pain. This can be very isolating and frightening for a child – who may well fail as a result, regardless of their innate intelligence and talents.

School is a place where your self-esteem can be raised to the roof or bashed pancake-flat. Few of us come out unscathed. Of course, school can be brilliant and great fun. It can also be hard going, leaving scars for life. School is a place of great social bonding, where deep friendships are made. It can also be a zoo, with bullying and gang-warfare. There is a lot of pressure to perform in class, pass exams and survive in the playground. Some children feel they can 'earn' self-esteem by pleasing teacher and appeasing friends. Most feel the need to belong and few feel they really do.

Going Up but Feeling Down

'Going up' from primary to secondary school can be exciting – and daunting. There are new rules to learn, new children to meet, new teachers to please and the exams get increasingly difficult and serious. Again, children often need a lot of understanding at this point; they might feel out of their depth, they might lose 'best-friends' and be bullied. This transition often means a child needs to process a lot of conflicting feelings, be listened to about anxieties, talk about successes, grieve over losing friends. They might even have nightmares and night sweats, or start bedwetting, all of which show a high level of fear. At this point, good co-operation between teachers and parents would be ideal, with plenty of time for a child to express his or her feelings.

1. Can you remember what it was like 'going up' from nursery to primary school, and primary to secondary school?

....

2. How was your self-esteem affected by school? Write down your thoughts on these issues in your notebook.

....

Peer Group Pressure

Being one-of-the-gang, is to belong. School is full of tests and challenges – and not just from teacher. Most of us can remember being 'dared' to smoke or face danger as part of an initiation ceremony. If you fail a 'dare', you are a 'divi', a 'dork', definitely 'uncool' and 'out'.

'I was petrified of school, and in particular of the other girls,' says Patti, now 43, and a mother of two, currently at secondary school. 'I was from a working-class family and got to Grammar School by passing the 11-plus exam. I was too good, and very unpopular because of it, so I started to be naughty to make friends. I had to steal money out of the teacher's purse, which I did; and smoke in the classroom, which I also did. I wanted desperately to belong.'

The lack of opportunity for young people to release their feelings in a supportive environment, is mainly to blame.

ADOLESCENCE: EXPERIMENTATION AND REBELLION

Adolescence is also a time for experimentation: finding out who you are, what you want, of becoming an individual in your own right. You also have little power and lots of dreams, wanting to lead an independent life while, frustratingly, not having the means to do so. Using addictions is also a way of managing the social pressures of maturing sexually, dating, trying to earn money, developing an independent lifestyle, while sorting out directions and careers. Addictions can be very attractive at this time, because they can also be forms of rebellion against the status quo, whereby you define who you are as different from your family. You might well start drinking, smoking, taking drugs in defiance of your parents' attitudes and behaviour.

Student/Trainee Life

Students are notorious for going wild and experimenting in every way – with drugs, alcohol, sex, clothes, music, ideas. Often, the first time a young person is unleashed from family ties is when they go to college, university or work abroad, so it can be both exciting, and scary. Trainees, on the other hand, might have to live at home because of lack of money, which can cause family friction. The social pressures on students and trainees can be enormous: learning to fit in, living alone or with new people, having to pay rent, bills and to cook and clean, managing money, falling in love, meeting tight study deadlines, sitting exams, learning new skills, handling competition, feeling inadequate and or worried about the future.

Jacob was the first in his family to go to university. 'I had such an unrealistic idea of what life would be like. I imagined it to be all sherry parties, with professors swanning about in gowns. So I was very shocked when I got there and found it was nothing like that.'

Jacob found it hard to break into social groups and, being Jewish, he also came up against anti-Semitism. In desperation, he resorted to watching two films a day and drinking beer every evening. 'I couldn't tell my parents how miserable I was, because they'd sacrificed so much for me to get there. I couldn't seem to make friends, or meet women, and I was too ashamed to go and talk to the college counsellor; that would have been stigma in itself. So I just drowned my sorrows as best I could.'

Jacob managed to work quite hard, but his isolated misery left a deep scar well into adulthood. To this day he can't visit his university town without all the terror and misery flooding back, still needing to be released. And he still buries himself in films and drink when the going gets tough.

Think about your own student/trainee days. Or perhaps you're a student now – what chemical and emotional addictions did/do you use to keep yourself going? When did/do you turn to them? Write down your experiences in your notebook.

....

....

WORK LIFE

If you work, you can spend most of your waking hours there. You can feel you see more of your colleagues than you do of your partner, family and friends. This is especially true if you work shifts and/or anti-social hours. Work obviously provides a means to live; it also provides a sense of self-worth and status. It teaches skills, stretches, satisfies, exhausts, or bores you, according to its nature and challenges. Work can also create all sorts of stresses and strains which can increase, rather than diminish, your addictions. This is because:

- Starting a new job is challenging. There is a lot to learn: systems, names, information; and there is a lot of emphasis on achievement and proving yourself. So you can feel pretty 'stressed-out'.

- Work 'culture' demands you be 'one-of-the-gang' in a similar way to school. You are a definite 'party-pooper' if you don't let your hair down and have a drink at Christmas or on someone's birthday or at a 'leaving do'. People can feel you are being 'superior' or holding back from being a 'team-player'.

- You need to be 'professional', which means not showing your feelings about either your domestic life or how you feel about the job. Being professional is very important, because a job obviously needs to be done effectively, and production would suffer if we all spent hours talking about our problems. But very often people get to work loaded down with worries about relationships, family, money, housing, children, health, further training and lack of promotion.

- The job might have its own internal difficulties, such as racial or sexual harassment, office politics or imminent redundancy. Or simply you might be bored because you are under-achieving, and/or are being badly managed. The bottling up of feelings can lead people to hit the pub, the gym or their partner hard after work, which is not the best way to deal with tension.

- The economic recession has created cutbacks: hours have got longer, staff fewer and pressures greater. Being over-stretched for a long period can lead to stress, which in turn can lead to increased use of everyday addictions. Workaholism – which is when you feel work is the only thing worth doing – wrecks marriages and health. It also creates and sustains other addictions (such as smoking, tranquillizers, alcohol, caffeine). If you only feel really alive when attached to your word-processor, lathe or mobile phone, then you are in trouble. That is when work crosses over from being a means to an end, to a dangerous end in itself.

- Holidays are defined as a break from work. On holiday we want to relax, reflect, slow down, spend time with our families, friends or even alone, recuperating from the stress of everyday life. But very often holidays become an excuse to use chemical addictions as a *means of winding down*. Of course, there is nothing wrong with the odd drink, special meal or ice-cream, but if you spend the whole holiday stuck to a bar stool then something's out of balance. There *are* pleasurable ways to relax without overspending, overeating, over drinking. (See Chapter 11: Meeting Your Physical Needs.)

1. If you work, which addictions do you use to keep going? Write down in your notebook how you start your day, what and when you drink, eat, snack on, etcetera.

   ....

2. What do you look for in a holiday? What addictions do you look forward to using?

   ....

UNEMPLOYMENT, REDUNDANCY

By no means has everyone got paid employment. And those who have may face the probability of redundancy daily. If you have already been made redundant, you may have been given a lump sum of money (which you may not know how to use) and you are faced with starting again, probably with a loss of status, possibly in midlife. Unemployment can be incredibly stressful, because:

- You have little or no money. Current rates of income support are extremely low and restrictions so numerous that the financial gap between being employed and being unemployed is now very wide. It is not a soft or easy option for a family of four or more to live on the dole. Without money it is difficult to eat well and virtually impossible to travel, go out, buy clothes and have fun as everything costs.

- You have little or no status. Contrary to popular belief, few people choose unemployment as a way of life. People gain status from their jobs, especially if their work makes a contribution to society, such as in nursing or teaching. But unemployed people don't have anything tangible to reflect themselves and their abilities.

- If you have been made redundant, you often suffer loss of status and it can be daunting to have to retrain at 40, 50 or even later. Worse, you may have to come to terms with no real prospect of ever working again at 40 plus.

- Relationships are under pressure, whether one or some, or all of your family is unemployed. There can be resentments, fears, changes in daily routine and chores, which fuel rows.

- It's isolating. You are not part of a group, not part of work life. You are floating in time, trying to get work, but getting nowhere fast. This does not mean that some people don't use their time very constructively, but if you are not part of an organization, no matter how small, it is hard to feel you belong to society.

- Unemployed people are often criticized for continuing to drink and smoke, or watch a lot of TV, while facing poverty and few prospects. But if you feel you have nothing to look forward to and you need to 'kill time', addictions become the 'treats' which brighten up a monotonous life. The problem with using addictions, is that the underlying painful emotions don't get handled, so your troubles can escalate.

- Some people do 'choose' to be unemployed because they scorn work. Often they are actually fearful of participating in society, so 'dropping out' is a way of not facing reality, and living in fantasy. This can be an isolating philosophy because it stems from the idea that you can truly 'opt out' and still claim social benefits. Addictions perpetuate the (phoney) belief that you can have a wonderful life by doing absolutely nothing at all.

So it's time to turn to your notebook again and jot down a few more observations.

1. If you're unemployed/have been made redundant, which addictions do you use and how?

....

2. Have your addictive habits changed since you stopped work?

....

EMERGING PATTERNS

This chapter has analysed how social pressures may have affected your getting addicted. Look back over the chapter and also see what you wrote down in your notebook after reading each section. Can you see any patterns emerging? Have your addictions increased or changed according to the amount or type of social pressure you have been under? Have they improved or even disappeared when your circumstances have changed?

Addictions are also the social glue that binds us together in everyday life, so it is to the role our relationships can play in getting us hooked, that we now turn in Chapter 5.

Chapter 5

———◦———

Facing Relationships

Relationships matter hugely; they are the fabric of everyday life, and they are built, extended, demolished and repaired all the time. As social beings we need all sorts of relationships: with family, friends, romantic and sexual, marital, or living together; with children, work colleagues, pets, with necessary professionals such as doctors, dentists, police, accountants, lawyers, with our God/s and Goddesses, and with ourselves. Relationships are where we live – and interact.

THE PAINS AND THE PLEASURES OF RELATIONSHIPS

Go into any pub, any mother and toddler group, listen in on any phonecall, eavesdrop during a tea-break at work, watch TV talk shows, read the gutterpress – and what are people talking about? – their relationships. And we ourselves are all constantly puzzling out our next moves, trying to reach each other and sort out misunderstandings, manipulating outcomes, negotiating agreements, second-guessing motives, assessing levels of commitment and safety. Relationships take up a lot of time and energy. You can spend hours worrying about them, improving them, arguing within them, agonizing as they collapse, trying to mend them, mourning their loss. You can reach moments of intense joy, closeness and trust and they can be wonderfully rewarding and supportive. They can also be utterly dreadful, leaving you miserable and spent.

GENDER DIFFERENCES AND RELATIONSHIP ISSUES

Walk into any newsagent and you will be faced by a wall of weekly and monthly women's magazines – boldly proclaiming on their front covers relationship issues:

- 'Spot the cheat: we've sussed the men most likely to stray' (*New Woman*).

- 'Should you have sex with your ex-lover? (Probably not, but we all do)' (*Cosmopolitan*).

- 'The lover and the loved: who's who in your relationship?' (*Options*).

- 'It's your fault: why do couples blame each other when the going gets tough?' (*Bella*).

- 'My husband fell in love with my brother' (*Woman*).

Typically, men's magazines largely ignore relationships, focusing more on so-called 'leisure activities', such as pornography; hobbies, such as computers, train-spotting; sports, body-beautiful and style. Even the 'new man'-ish glossy magazines, like *GQ* and *Esquire*, have endless articles on Arnold Schwarzenegger, female 'pin ups' like Pamela Anderson, plus more of the usual 'male' diet of sport, hobbies, fashion, travel and cars. But there are signs of change here. These two headlines appeared on the cover of a *GQ* issue: 'Are you man enough to sleep with your boss?' and 'Male infertility: do your sperm count?'

However, relationship issues are more usually restricted to the occasional light-hearted piece, such as 'How To Dump Your Girlfriend' (*FHM*).

Oddly, men's glossy magazines don't often have 'agony uncles', although it's well known that men read and write to the agony aunts featured in women's magazines. Does this mean men can't own up to needing help with their relationship problems? Or do they regard it as being 'woman's work', along with cleaning, cooking, child-rearing, and so on? Clearly, men want good relationships, but perhaps they still shun 'emotional literacy' because it is 'wimpish navel-gazing'. Of course, there are some men who meet in men's groups and talk about feelings, but they are a rare breed. Even the 'radical', 'new men's' magazine *Achilles Heel* avoids personal 'show and tell' articles, favouring political and intellectual analysis.

Lesbian/Gay/Bisexual Relationships

Most mainstream women's and men's magazines make an assumption that everyone is heterosexual, so the relationship difficulties faced by lesbian women, gay men and bisexuals are virtually never discussed – except by the occasional token article. Because of this editorial censorship, it is very difficult to get any intelligent, informed discussion addressing real issues. And in particular, it is extremely difficult to write about addiction in lesbian/gay/bisexual relationships. This is because it is often tacitly implied in mainstream journals that to be lesbian/gay/bisexual is, in itself, a problem, thereby putting homosexual writers on the defensive.

Yet sexuality is not a fixed thing, and within a lifetime, people may experience being actively heterosexual, gay, bisexual, lesbian and/or celibate, so magazines should bear this in mind when making assumptions about their readership. Because of the stigma still attached to being gay/lesbian/bisexual, there are few places where the issue of addictive relationships and homosexuality can be discussed without falling into a polarized debate about 'for' and 'against'. This perpetuates a great deal of isolation for gay/lesbian/bisexual people, and ignorance in society at large – as well as fear of homophobia in people who are thinking about 'coming out'.

ADDICTIVE RELATIONSHIPS

The worst kinds of relationships are addictive ones. This is because people get trapped in them, like insects under glass, unable to breathe, move, think or manoeuvre. Sometimes they get squashed altogether. Most confusing of all, an addictive relationship usually has the 'Feel Good Factor'. You can feel wonderfully alive, totally worshipped, sexually insatiable, amazingly helpful, that you 'were made for each other', joined at the hip, that this is 'the love of your life', on an exciting roller-coaster of passion, that you have so much in common, etcetera. Usually this is a deadly cocktail of desperation and isolation, mixed with love and sex addiction and a dash of fear to give it a bite.

Cause and Effect

If you have come from an unhappy family, then the likelihood is you could find it hard to make satisfying relationships. If you haven't experienced healthy give and take, as well as the rough and tumble of family life, while being loved and cared for at the same time, it will obviously be very difficult to create this for yourself in adult life. This is especially true if your family harboured addiction within it. For instance, children brought up in alcoholic families find it difficult to trust, and to talk about themselves. They feel guilty, over-responsible and have low self-esteem. They seldom feel loved; they feel everything's very black or white, can be melodramatic, hate chaos, but yet create it in their own lives by falling in love with the 'wrong' people, who often have similar addictions to those of their parent(s). These adults feel they never were children, because the burden of family problems was inappropriately placed on their shoulders far too early. They may have been forced to be care-takers, have lived in pretence and squalor, and have been deeply frightened of, and perhaps hated by, the very people who are supposed to look after and care for them.

So the root of addictive relationships usually lies in our experience of early and family life (as we saw in Chapter 3). At the same time, the driving emotional force is our frozen needs: those real needs which were never met, or inadequately met, when we needed them to be. The unreleased pain attached to our frozen needs is precisely what keeps us wanting. Many of us are still looking (in vain) for the mothers and fathers we never had. We carry deep wells of loneliness, caverns of emptiness, which we try to fill with romance, love and sex. We're always looking for 'the one' who will make a difference. We also try to replace people we have lost through death, separation or the end of a relationship.

We can become obsessed with looks, clothes, habits, preferences of our 'loved ones' – which often, on closer inspection, remind us of our long lost mum and dad who never loved us enough, or approved enough, or made us feel special. Or maybe they loved us too much, swamped us with their needs, even sexually abused and beat us, all factors which can lead to relationship addiction. We are continually trying to get it right and 'win' with someone in the present, as if this will change or compensate for the past, when we got it wrong and 'lost'. It won't.

As we saw in Chapter 2, frozen needs can never be filled; no matter how hard we try. All we can do is face up to this fact and do the grieving, talking, raging and shaking necessary to help us accept it. For most of us this is far too painful to consider, so we continue to throw ourselves, lemming-like, into a succession of relationships, trying to meet those frozen needs. Each time, we can end up miserable, disappointed, frustrated, embittered, bashed and rejected, saying 'never again'. Yet, after a painful period of mourning we are dusted down and ready for more punishment, and we go steaming in again.

Types of Addictive Relationships

There are several different types of addictive relationships, and some contain more than one element of addiction. Family relationships, friendships, and work relationships can be addictive, although we tend to focus more on sexual/romantic relationships when we think about addiction. So what kinds of addictive relationship are there?

Relationships based on addiction.   If you have a chemical and or emotional addiction, say, to alcohol, sex, gambling, food, and/or TV-watching, it can be very attractive to find someone who will do it with you – or at least approve of *you* doing it. People collude with each other by agreeing to over-eat, overwork, have addictive sex, spend too much, drink till they fall over. This collusion relieves feelings of guilt and shame, of having to justify and explain anti-social and/or self-abusive behaviour, and it creates a bonding, a camaraderie. You can end up in a downward spiral, because neither of you is able to counter the other; instead you egg each other on. The experience of doing it together becomes central to the relationship, forming a common language, and fond 'over-the-top' memories.

One woman in her sixties boasted to me during a counselling session that she had found the 'perfect partner' and was having the 'best sex of her life'. In fact, she was putting up with physical violence from a 40-year-old 'gigolo', who joined in with her in compulsive sex, excessive drinking, smoking and drug-taking. He was also stealing her money. Yet, she was willing to suffer the battering and thieving in exchange for a drug-mate.

The test of this kind of relationship, like all addictive relationships, is what happens if one partner gives up the addiction or modifies it. There is usually a lot of aggression on both sides, and the relationship disintegrates, unable to take the strain of one partner becoming 'clean'. People no longer seem attractive to each other as a consequence; they can suddenly seem very boring, or draining.

Using addiction as emotional blackmail.   This can work in two ways: either one person nags the other to join in on the chemical/emotional addiction: 'Go on, don't be boring. You don't know till you've tried it. Live a little, let your hair down. If you *really* loved me, you'd do it,' and so on. Alternatively, if the addictive behaviour is a major character flaw in one partner, it can elevate the 'sober' partner to dizzy heights of bullying perfection: 'You should be more like me, I know best,' and so on.

In the first case, the addicted person can't bear to be alone with their particular addiction. In fact, they usually feel very ashamed and are deeply relieved if they can get the other partner to 'crack'. It normalizes their own behaviour – if their friend/partner does it, it must be all right. In the second case, the sober partner/friend uses sobriety as a stick to bludgeon and manipulate the addicted one. It can just be an excuse for another form of abuse. In fact, they are both locked into an addictive relationship – one of control and be controlled (see also Codependency below).

Addiction is being used to exert emotional blackmail in both cases and, again, if one partner changes their role, it will change the balance of power and the relationship will probably die.

Addiction as a smokescreen. If your relationship is in trouble and there are deep-seated problems that neither of you is facing upfront, then you can use addiction as a smokescreen. This means you may try desperately to 'have a good time', by, say, having expensive meals, buying pricey gifts, drinking and eating too much together. It is a way of the orchestra playing on as the ship sinks. Eventually, something usually happens whereby both partners/friends have to stop and think.

One couple tried to mend their relationship by cooking more and more elaborate meals for each other. They had a round of dinner parties, and went out for candlelit suppers all the time. Eventually, they both put on a lot of weight, ceased fancying each other and stopped making love. When the woman finally said she was going to lose weight and wanted to diet – they rowed. It was a bitter, volcanic fight, which rumbled on for weeks. All the suppressed resentments and problems came to the surface – because she had decided to take a different (and more threatening) direct course of action. In this situation, you need to mirror each other and take the new steps together – or the relationship will fail.

Codependency. This is where one person is addicted to another with an addiction. Most commonly, it is associated with alcohol, but can be about other chemical or emotional addictions. Codependents base their whole lives on martyrdom. Their one topic of conversation is the other one's problem; drinking/smoking/drug-taking/overworking/overspending. They worry about it day and night, phone helplines and counsellors 'on behalf' of the other person, and, like the 'emotional blackmail' type of addictive relationship, spend a lot of time making the other person feel guilty, worthless, and beholden.

In fact, codependency is a desperate need to control someone else because you, yourself, feel so out of control. If you focus on someone else's problems, then your own apparently diminish. But it is an illusion. All you are doing is putting the headlights on the overtly-addicted person and feeling squeaky-clean yourself as a result.

Often, when the overtly-addicted person gives up or cuts down their addiction from their own volition, the relationship begins to falter. The focus swings towards the codependent partner, who doesn't like having attention turned on them, because they don't want anyone to see the cracks in their carefully constructed façade. They can no longer be completely good, because the other person is no longer very bad. This kind of relationship gets extremely uncomfortable at this point and, again, may well disintegrate because there is nothing left at the centre.

Relationships based on domination/submission. Who has got the upper hand can be a constant, unspoken competition in these addictive relationships. Someone's got to win, so someone's got to lose. Sometimes a relationship can start out with one person 'on top', only to swing around so that the other takes control. There is always a winner and a loser; one jubilant, the other bleeding on the ropes. Yet, both have usually been deeply hurt and can't love or trust. Sometimes it is a 'victim' falling in love with a 'bastard'; there may be sado-masochism in the bedroom or there may be emotional sado-masochism, or both. The tacit agreement is that one partner must dominate, so the other must submit.

In both cases, there is usually some history of sexual and/or physical abuse, and/or neglect. The sado-masochistic practice is an indirect way of trying to get to and release the pain. However, because it is often a re-enactment of the original hurt, it can create more distress than it relieves (even if you were beaten as a child and are now doing the beating). The 'Feel Good Factor' comes into play here as both partners can defend sado-masochism on the basis that it brings pleasure and pain (there is a thin line between these sensual experiences anyway). Sometimes one partner wishes to break out of this kind of violent relationship, but feels too hooked to change it from within. The only option can become one of having to escape altogether with your life, because once you have crossed such a relationship rubicon it is virtually impossible to go back.

Obsessive love. This is a major form of relationship addiction. Usually one partner is 'fatally attracted' to the point of obsession, while the object of desire remains indifferent. Often the whole relationship is mere fantasy in the mind of the adorer. Obsessive love is always based on frozen needs, an old desire to possess that which cannot be possessed.

Inevitably, the obsession is a way of covering up deep emotional hurts which, if the obsessed person stopped to consider long enough, they'd probably feel. So the obsession is like an anaesthetic, numbing out everything, bar the object of obsession.

Of course, if the object of desire becomes a real person, the worshipper is often quickly disillusioned. The adored-one has faults: spots, erratic or painful periods, is gauche or ill-mannered, has the wrong accent – in fact, will not solve all the problems or meet all the frozen needs of the adorer. So deep depression follows disappointment, sometimes with an urge to turn to other addictions, like alcohol, self-mutilation, even suicide.

Assessing Your Own Relationships

What about you? Do you recognize any of these addictive relationships in your own life? If so, which? How do you feel about it? Write down your responses in your notebook.

....

....

You *can* tackle addictive relationships if you want to get off the hook, but, as with all addictions, you have to decide you *want* to first (see Chapter 8: Making the Break, and Chapter 9: Being Your Own Parent). You then need to identify and try to meet your own real relationship needs instead. This is discussed further in Chapter 10: Meeting Your Emotional Needs, Chapter 12: Meeting Your Sexual Needs and Chapter 13: Meeting Your Social Needs.

HANDLING RELATIONSHIPS

Relationships go through all sorts of stages and forms, from casual acquaintance to marriage to obsessive love, and back. It can often be difficult for both partners to agree, exactly, what status a relationship has, because:

- You may find it hard to communicate your thoughts and feelings about a relationship to the other person involved, because you're frightened of being too vulnerable, or saying something offensive and hurting feelings. Or you may be embarrassed, fearing to seem too keen, getting in too deep, fearing conflict.

- You may find it hard to listen to the other person in a relationship with you because you fear rejection, criticism, thereby making you feel hurt, or their being over-keen, over-committed to you, making you feel guilty, or restricted in making or developing other relationships.

- You may be confused about exactly what you want in a relationship, and feel it's better to avoid having one altogether, or keep a relationship very limited to avoid possible pain.

Handling Conflict

Addictions are often used to handle conflict in relationships; people can turn to drink, prostitution, drugs, spending money, TV-watching, to ward off having to face reality. Some women have problems with establishing emotional boundaries, often due to having grown up with controlling, dominating or intrusive parents, or having experienced some form of abuse (sexual and/or physical). In such circumstances they haven't learned where 'you' begins and 'I' ends. If *you* have no boundaries, you may be inappropriately over-intimate in relationships and you may expect your partners to be the same. You may be impatient or bored with the gradual growth of trust, closeness and commitment inherent in healthy relationships. You will probably want total commitment from day one and be very disappointed when a friend or lover seems to be less interested and/or committed.

A healthy balance in relationships would probably be to have no rigid barriers, blocking intimacy, but rather definite boundaries, which allowed relationships to develop to appropriate levels of intimacy over time. All too few of us experience this healthy balance, however, which is why we scour the media and self-help books for help.

Relationship Breakdown

When relationships break down, months, even years, of pent-up pain can come flying out of an emotional Pandora's Box. People can feel so hurt, insecure, confused and abandoned that they turn to their favourite addictions for 'security'. Most of us know someone who, after a separation or divorce, has turned to alcohol for solace. Others embark on a succession of affairs 'on the rebound', in a desperate, and usually futile, attempt to boost their confidence. Whatever your particular resources may be, when a relationship breaks down you are in a very vulnerable state.

Poor communication. Relationships usually break down because we haven't been able to be as direct as we needed to be in communicating our feelings, grievances, resentments, thoughts, desires, and fears, during the relationship. In fact, breakdown usually occurs when you reach the pinnacle of a mountain of misunderstanding. If you can keep channels of communication open during a relationship, there's usually a better chance of resolving problems as they occur – or at least airing them – so you never have to climb too far up the mountain.

Mourning the break. While it is totally understandable that people turn to addictions to handle a relationship breakdown, such activities never have positive long-term results. You may gain temporary relief from the pain of separation, but you can end up on the Addictive Treadmill, trapped by an endless cycle of addiction-induced 'ups' and 'downs'. It is necessary to face the fact that the relationship is over (if it is), and mourn appropriately while getting support from friends, family and colleagues. Relationship breakdown can feel utterly devastating, especially if it was a long-term relationship and children are involved. It can be even harder, if one, or both, partners have a relationship/s with a third, or even fourth party. The period of mourning will depend upon the length, depth and nature of the relationship, and people often underestimate the time needed to grieve and recover. (A rough estimate is one or two years at *least* for a committed long-term relationship. It also depends on whether you were left or did the leaving: the leaver usually recovers faster because they were 'in charge'.)

RELATIONSHIP COUNSELLING/ THERAPY

Some couples go to a counsellor or therapist when their relationship is dissolving. Or, just one partner may seek personal counselling support. Sometimes, a whole family (including young children) will go into therapy. It can be extremely helpful to air problems with a third party who is objective and trained to help everyone communicate more clearly with each and every other member. It is never a sign of failure to seek outside help; rather, it is a courageous step and a sign of hope, although some people (especially men) still feel there's a stigma attached to asking for psychological help.

Many relationships and families have been pulled back from the brink of total breakdown just by having a chance to air long-held misunderstandings and resentments. Relationship breakdowns are very daunting and exhausting, and people usually are desperate to salvage what they can after years of emotional investment.

Have you experienced relationship breakdown? What happened? How did you feel? Did you turn to addictions to 'cope'? What was your worst experience? What did you learn about you and relationships? Write down your answers in your notebook.

....

....

Your Support Network

Some people are immensely supported by loving families, which provide good models for the rest of their relationships. Others may not have experienced much tender, loving care at home, or may have been none too happily adopted, fostered, or surrogated, and in consequence may find it hard to create their own close family. Some people make deliberate choices to sever ties with their blood-relations, and create their own 'family' networks with like-minded people.

Take a moment to think: which are your closest relationships? Who matters to you? Supports you? Do you have best friends? Spouse/partner? Children? Imagine you are the hub of a wheel, with spokes sticking out in all directions. In your notebook, draw the spokes different lengths according to how close you feel to each person and put their name beside the relevant spoke.

Here's an example:

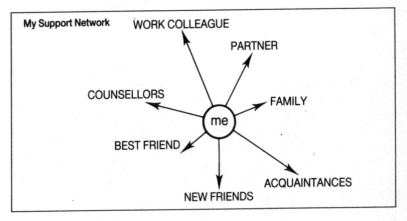

This is your support network. Whenever you are feeling isolated and that nobody cares, get out your notebook and look at your support network – and don't forget to keep it up to date by adding new relationships as they become established; and deleting others as they erode.

Of course, from time to time we all experience crises, whether a relationship breakdown, the death of someone important to us, accident great or small, financial failure, redundancy, serious, even terminal, illness; or you might be involved in a 'disaster' such as a bomb or major fire. How crises can cause you to get hooked to one or more addictions is the subject of Chapter 6.

Chapter 6

■—○—■

Facing Crises

I have certainly had my fair share of crises: handling other peoples' suicide attempts; getting run over by a lorry; losing beloved friends through fatal accidents or illnesses; handling a stranger's heart-attack and a car crash; being heart-broken by ruthless lovers; being made redundant; going on strike; experiencing separation and divorce. I know how devastating these experiences can be – and also how everyday addictions can often seem the only answer to excruciating emotional and physical pain. I've also counselled many clients who had turned to various forms of addiction as a way of handling their own crises.

AVOIDANCE THROUGH ADDICTION

The time just after a crisis is when we are at our most vulnerable; and that is when addictions can all too easily take hold. If you feel the urge to blot out the pain, it is very tempting to reach for the bottle, the pills, or the video. Reaching for addictions is a bad idea.

As you have already seen, you can get hooked on to the Addictive Treadmill and end up feeling bad, feeling worse, feeling absolutely terrible. Addictions don't solve your problems and, in fact, often create more problems (for instance, impairing your judgement, which can lead to yet another accident/crisis). It can also make you feel you can only ever cope with a crisis with the 'help' of your chemical/emotional addictions. This further undermines your confidence in coping by relying on yourself or others.

POST-TRAUMATIC SHOCK DISORDER

Crises nearly always happen when you least expect them. You can be sailing along in your life, feeling pretty good about your job, your relationships, yourself when, wham, something happens, completely out of the blue and you are floored. Crises are renowned for their bad timing, as Josie found out:

'It was a beautiful summer's evening, I was having a great time with friends and we'd just been to see a very funny film. I had just changed jobs and was very excited because I'd been offered an amazing project and was to start work on it the next day. We were walking down the street, chatting about the film, when a motorbike suddenly careered round the corner, up on to the pavement and pinned me against the wall. I screamed and passed out. When I came to, minutes later, the lower half of my body hurt like hell and I knew instantly that something serious was wrong. I couldn't move my legs and I was in utter agony. None of my friends was hurt, and I was thankful for that, but in an odd sort of way it also made me feel very alone.'

In fact, Josie's legs and pelvis were broken (the bike rider was unhurt), and she spent the next four months in traction, in hospital, followed by three months of intensive physiotherapy. Josie's accident threw her plans completely – and she missed out on the project she had been so excited about. After her accident, Josie went through the 'normal' emotional reaction to crisis – what is now commonly known as 'post-traumatic shock disorder'.

The Symptoms of Post-traumatic Shock Disorder

Going numb. People often feel they are floating in unreality, or in a dream-like state; feeling very odd and detached. This is a natural response to fear, when the body releases 'natural' biochemical painkillers and tranquillizers (called endorphins). Their purpose is to stop us putting ourselves in further danger, or being completely overwhelmed by fear – or anxiety (you can also feel like this when under severe stress).

Feeling anxious (yet more fear). When the numbness wears off, there is often a rush of adrenalin, more blood is directed to the muscles and you breathe faster, taking in more oxygen. Your heart pounds, your hands and knees shake, you may pant and/or feel breathless, as though you can't get enough air. You can feel highly anxious, your mind in emotional turmoil as you struggle with thoughts, such as: 'How am I going to cope? Who is going to feed the cat? Am I going to die? Why me? How long will it take to get better? What am I going to tell my boss/family/friends/spouse/family?'

Can't sleep, but feel exhausted. The stress of a crisis pumps yet more chemicals into the bloodstream which put you on 'red alert'. Sleeplessness is a way of staying 'vigilant' in readiness for the next attack. Exhaustion, even if you have not done anything particularly physical, or mentally stretching, results from staying vigilant. You might feel that life is happening in slow motion. The hours drag by, your limbs feel heavy, you have headaches, and aches and pains in your legs, arms, hands, stomach, which nothing seems to ease. You can feel apathetic, so that you 'can't be bothered' to wash or change your clothes, or concentrate on anything, or even watch TV.

Disturbed sleep/dreams/nightmares. You probably drop off to sleep from time to time, but may jerk awake suddenly, feeling very panicked. You may have disturbing dreams or repetitive nightmares; in consequence, you may fear sleeping.

But, in fact, this is the mind's way of trying to absorb what has happened. You may 'remember' things in your dreams which have been blocked off by shock. You may wake up sweating, shaking and screaming – but these unpleasant reactions are all part of the natural emotional release explained in Chapter 2.

Slowed-down/confused thinking – accompanying exhaustion or lack of sleep – is often a feeling that your brain isn't working properly. It seems to have slowed down and/or is confused. People lose or forget things all the time during this phase: put a pot to boil on the stove and forget all about it, dial phone-numbers and can't remember whom they're calling or why. If it happens to you, you can feel as if your brain is covered in treacle. You can't follow what people are saying to you and they have to repeat everything several times. You can't make sense of the simplest things. This can be very frightening and you may even feel that you're going 'mad'. You are not. It is a completely natural response to shock, and you will eventually feel better.

Can't eat (or swallow). You can feel sick and full up with post-traumatic shock, and food can look revolting. You might even stop eating altogether for a day or so. Well-meaning friends and family may try to force you to eat, but you just can't swallow. Often you can feel overpowered by other peoples' anxiety about your eating. If you do eat, you may throw up or suffer bad indigestion – this is all due to your high levels of stress.

Obsessive thinking. You may find yourself telling the story of your particular crisis over and over and over, or thinking about it obsessively. You may keep repeating the scene in your mind and trying to change the ending, to a positive outcome. This kind of mental preoccupation is completely normal. As with nightmares and dreams (above), it is your mind's way of coming to terms with what has happened. The painful emotion surrounding the event is making it hard for your brain to assimilate what has occurred, and the obsessive thinking is a way of trying to understand something very frightening.

Depending on the degree of trauma, this preoccupation may last just a few hours or days, or very much longer if not treated – you may still have 'flashbacks' long afterwards, when something in your everyday life reminds you of the original event.

Changed behaviour. You may change your habits and routines completely in response to a crisis. You may cease to drive, and only watch TV, or you may wear different clothes or stop going to work. You may well disturb those around you because you're so different. Maybe you can't laugh at anything, or you burst into tears a lot, or you feel frightened of things you usually take in your stride. This temporary withdrawal and/or strange behaviour is due to shock – and may be a way of protecting yourself from any further shocks.

Grief. Once numbness wears off, you may start feeling very weepy at the slightest thing. Again, this is a natural response to needing to process the grief of the event. You may cry a lot when you go to bed and when you wake up, because you suddenly remember what's happened and there's nothing to distract you. You may wake up and cry in the night, because you can't go back to sleep, and feel lonely and desperate.

Anger. Along with grieving (usually after a good bout of crying), you can begin to feel very angry. A feeling of 'why me?' can envelop you in bitterness. Everything looks bleak and you feel furious that you have been singled out for bad luck. You may begin to hate other people who seem so happy, relaxed and unhurt. You may focus your hate on someone else in or around the crisis, who seems to have got off lightly. You may also turn the hate on yourself, obsessively thinking you should have done something different – and how then it could have all been avoided.

Shame and guilt. Grief and anger is usually accompanied by shame and guilt, so that your emotions are in turmoil. You can feel that you caused the crisis, that you got off too lightly (especially if someone else died). The shame arises from feeling self-consciously uncomfortable, and the guilt is about feeling morally at odds with yourself. These feelings need to be dealt with, so that you do not turn your hatred on yourself and hurt yourself further. (See Chapters 1 and 2.)

Depression.   Bouts of depression usually follow crises. You feel a mixture of all of the feelings already discussed above: lethargy, tearfulness, anger, shame, guilt, lack of appetite or sleeplessness. You may withdraw from usual social contact or take time off work. Depression is basically anger turned in on yourself – it may last a few hours, days, weeks, months – or in severe cases – much longer. (See Chapter 10 for ways to prevent this happening to you.)

Vulnerable to illness.   After a crisis your immune system is weakened, especially if negative feelings are not dealt with. You can be very vulnerable to viral infections or worse, because you are not eating or sleeping normally and are feeling depressed. Sometimes you welcome illness simply to get some relief – at least it provides a reason for retreating into bed and hoping the world will go away. It can also be a cry for help.

Suicidal.   You can get suicidal feelings after a severe crisis, especially if you feel you were in some way to blame. Such feelings arise out of a sense of worthlessness, hopelessness and powerlessness. You may feel you want to hurt yourself further, that you don't deserve to live (or, indeed, that there is nothing to live for). But remember: suicidal feelings *don't* last forever, even though they feel as if they will at the time. (See Chapter 11.)

Isolation.   During and after a crisis you can feel very isolated, that no-one else really understands what has happened to you, and that they don't really care. This feeling of isolation can be so overpowering that it can cause you to turn to addictions to numb out the pain. Try to resist this. Be assured that this feeling is completely normal in crises and it *will* pass, especially if you can talk about it to someone.

FACING UP TO CRISES

Even if you are usually a pretty good 'coper', crises can throw you into complete turmoil. And life will have its crises – it can't possibly always be problem free, where everything always goes according to plan. Life is unpredictable and sometimes messy, and in fact, you can learn a lot about yourself, other people and the world through handling crises (or at least surviving them). Take comfort from the fact that every crisis survived will add to your confidence and ability to survive the next one, especially if you've healed emotionally.

If you have begun to face and release your feelings (see Chapter 2) and are becoming more emotionally literate, you can actually use crises to deepen your knowledge about how emotions work. Wisdom, compassion and deeper human connection can be an unexpected bonus from an experience which can look, at the outset, as though it has ruined your life. Tell yourself that addiction is *not* the answer to a crisis – as understandable as the temptation to succumb may be – remember that it is only a way of short-changing yourself in the long term. You can make a drama out of a crisis – or you can use it to become a more rounded and compassionate human being, and stay off the Addictive Treadmill.

Finally, before we move on to examining how to resist and overcome addiction by learning *how* to meet your real needs, in Chapter 7 let us look at one last way in which you can get hooked.

Chapter 7

―■○■―

Facing Oppression

To help you understand the power of oppression – and some of the ways in which it can cause people to turn to addictions for solace, I'd like to introduce you to some people who have fought to reshape their lives.

MAEVE O'CONNELL: NEVER A CHILD

'My mother started treating me like a grown up when I was three and a half years old. I had to do chores and look after my younger sister. Three more babies came and I looked after them, too, so there was never time to be a child. I got beat around the head by my mum when she got drunk and lost control, and I was beat up by my two elder brothers – in the presence of my parents – who did nothing about it. My dad was also a heavy drinker, unavailable emotionally, as well as physically. I didn't realize at the time how hard it all was. I just tried to be a good little girl, helping mum, trying to rescue the family – although I remember always thinking, "I can't wait to grow up".'

Maeve is 38, Irish, working-class and raised as a Catholic in Eire. She is now intent on getting off the hook from alcoholism, codependency and sex addiction.

BILL SMITH: ALL BOTTLED UP

'I was addicted to heroin from 13 to 19 years of age. I'm now 36. I stopped using heroin when I fell in love with Diane, who's now my wife. I stopped the only way I knew how – I gritted my teeth, clenched my fists, held everything in, and stayed drunk and stoned on marijuana for six weeks. It hurt. It was agony. I told nobody, not even Diane for a while. All my conditioning told me that was how men got through bad times. Having been out of control for six years, it seemed absolute control was the only answer. I'm glad I kicked it – I later gave up drinking and smoking too – but all the guilt, shame, self-loathing and disgust I still held in – like a real man.'

Bill, aged 49, English; working-class, raised in London's East End – beginning to release the bottled-up emotions and heal after six years of heroin and a lifetime of alcohol and nicotine.

LEAH THORNE: MAKE-UP SURVIVOR

'I was about nine years old when I first wore make-up. My mother had told me I looked 'verpischt' (a Yiddish word meaning something like 'washed out'). She proceeded to smear pink lipstick on my cheeks and mouth and I quickly got the message that with make-up on, I was prettier, looked healthier and was more acceptable to the world. Over the next 32 years I became addicted to make-up. I've used it as a prop to feel better about myself, and as armour against the pain I feel as a result of the ways I'm mistreated as a Jewish woman in this society.'

Leah, aged 43, Jewish/British working-class, getting off the hook from her make-up addiction (she also leads 'Face the World' workshops for women wanting to do the same; see 'Help' section at end of book).

VERA CUMMINS: COMPULSIVE EATER

'We never had enough food to eat in my family and, as a consequence, I'm now struggling with a food addiction. I come from a large, poor, family, who came to Britain from Barbados in the 1950s. I am now three stone overweight – a big woman. I'm particularly hooked on 'baby foods', such as strained fruit, chocolate pudding, yoghurt and ice-cream – in fact, all the things I never got as a child. I never seem to feel full and if I buy these foods I stuff them in very fast. They don't hit the back of my throat. I do it in secret, afraid I will get found out. I feel so guilty. Yet, I know my eating is linked to the survival eating patterns of poor people. I learned to stuff myself this way to stay alive as a child.'

Vera, aged 51, Barbadian/British, beginning to face up to the roots of her compulsive eating.

PETE DAVIES: A STOLEN CHILDHOOD

'I'm writing to you from prison, where I'm serving a sentence for stealing. I used to steal from all kinds of shops, I even stole money from friends, convincing myself "they" didn't play fair, or, "I found it, so it's mine", or "they're rich, so they don't need it". I recently started getting "flashbacks" to being about two years old, when my father started molesting me. He did it for years. I started stealing from him around that time. He told me I was "wonderful" and he loved me, but I felt it was a lie. I've felt all my life that no-one really cares for me – only about what they could get from me. I felt I had to be the best, look the best, to get approval. Then they would love me. So I started stealing, to get the best for myself. But deep inside I was hoping someone would catch me and help me stop. After all, I just want to be loved for being myself.'

Pete, aged 24, working-class, from North of England. Now receiving counselling help for sexual abuse, having completed his prison sentence for burglary.

What All These People Have in Common

Oppression. While growing up they all experienced some form of deprivation, prejudice, mistreatment, lack of vital resources (food, money, clothes), abuse, hardship, due to belonging to one or more oppressed groups (for example, Irish, female, working-class).

Addiction. All developed addictions in response to not getting their real needs (for love, affection, attention, safety, shelter, warmth, validation, nourishment) met in childhood. They all have low self-esteem and feel isolated and unlovable.

OPPRESSION AND OUTDATED PREJUDICES

Our culture has a pecking order which assigns value to human beings according to the groups we belong to. In order for someone to be 'on top', someone else has to be underneath. It is an unfair system based on outdated prejudices. For instance, it says:

- Men are superior to women.
- White people are worth more than black people.
- Working-class people are less intelligent than middle- or upper-class people.
- Adults are better than young people.
- Disabled people are less valuable than able-bodied people.

This oppressive system needs some people to feel worse or 'bad', so that others can feel better or 'good'.

We imbibe ideas about our worth from pre-birth onwards. Beliefs about our value are then further reinforced through family, school, work, and other formative experiences, as we have seen in earlier chapters. If you come from a background of hardship, prejudice, violence, denial and addiction – that way of life becomes 'normal'. If you are used to harsh treatment, it is difficult to treat yourself (and others) with love, tenderness and respect, even if that is what you secretly crave.

Who is Oppressed?

Many people are oppressed literally from birth; many more gradually join their number for a variety of circumstances – most of which are difficult if not impossible to avoid.

- Women are oppressed through sexism (men are also harmed by sexism).

- Black people, and ethnic minority people are oppressed through racism.

- Disabled people are oppressed through able-bodiedism.

- Young people are oppressed through adultism.

- Older people are oppressed through ageism.

- Lesbian women/gay men/bisexuals are oppressed through sexism and homophobia.

- Working-class people are oppressed by classism (middle- and upper-class people are also harmed by classism).

Oppression may also be suffered by artists, prisoners, lone parents, non-English speakers, people with particular religious beliefs, such as Catholics, Jews; people of Celtic heritage, such as the Welsh, Irish, Scottish, and Cornish. This list is not exhaustive – can you think of any more? Write them down.

....

....

Are You Oppressed?

You may never have thought of some of the above groups as being oppressed before. But are *you* oppressed? It can feel quite disturbing to think of yourself as belonging to an oppressed group – so you may not want to face it. But as we saw earlier the first step towards overcoming addictions is to face up to where your addictions began and how they continue to operate in your life. Oppression might be yet another aspect of your life which you have not considered as linking to addiction before. So take a moment to think about yourself and the groups you belong to – write them down in your notebook.

....

....

Multiple Oppression

Some people experience 'multiple oppression' because they fit into more than one oppressed group. The reality of life, if you belong to several oppressed groups, can be very hard. As we saw at the beginning of this chapter, if you are Irish, female, working-class, Catholic and poor, as is Maeve, you can suffer from the impact of five different sorts of oppression, all of which are telling you simultaneously that you are worthless, stupid, ignorant, bad, etcetera.

If *you* belong to more than one oppressed group, then you are probably experiencing multiple oppression (even if you can't feel it). This means your self-esteem is probably taking a battering from more than one type of prejudice. It is very hard to feel good about yourself when all the signs say you have no reason to feel good.

Internalized Oppression

Internalized oppression means believing the misinformation which exists about your group, and applying it to yourself. For instance, sexism says women are stupid gossips. If you are a woman and you believe that about yourself or other women, then you have internalized that oppression. It works in subtle ways, too. Women are constantly judged according to appearance: size, shape, colouring, etcetera. Internalized oppression makes women assess themselves and each other all the time as if they were looking through the eyes of the oppressor. Any back-biting that goes on between people in the same group is usually based on internalized oppression – as members of a group are set up against each other to compete for the crumbs society throws at them. Also, if you step out of line and start acting as if you were no longer oppressed, then you start being called 'uppity', 'you're getting above your station', or being 'too pushy'. So you can't win either way – or so it seems. Internalized oppression, whatever its nature, undermines personal confidence and power.

ADDICTION – AND ITS CONNECTION WITH OPPRESSION

Addiction and oppression go together because addictions are based on self-abuse and reinforce the idea that you're worthless, unimportant. They also anaesthetize the emotional and physical pain caused by being oppressed. Once you are in this highly vulnerable state your addictions can often become an 'entrance fee' to your oppressed group. Some examples are: young people 'belonging' by sniffing glue or taking Ecstasy, black people smoking marijuana, working-class women playing Bingo, working-class men drinking beer, and so on.

Don't forget – addictions are based on:

- Having low self-esteem.

- Feeling isolated.

- Feeling unloved and unlovable.

- Self-loathing/self-hatred.

- Believing you deserve to be abused.

Addictions as Allies

Oddly, your addictions have probably been your allies at some times during your life. By protecting you from facing reality they have enabled you to survive what probably would have been excruciating pain. If there were no more positive resources available to help you release your pain, your addictions have probably been necessary anaesthetics.

For instance, Ben, a northern, working class Catholic, came to me about his compulsive eating, but soon was telling me about a violent, deprived childhood, where his drunken father would beat him with a riding crop for no real reason, except usual boyish naughtiness, such as being noisy. Everyone could see the boy's painful humiliation because the punishment was carried out in front of an open window. Yet no adult came to stop it. Ben felt abandoned and betrayed, even by his mother, who was either in the next room or stood and watched. Had Ben had an ally at that point, to step in and take the whip away and to hold him close and let him scream, cry and rage – then these incidents would not have left such lasting, deep scars. But no-one stepped in, no-one listened to him as he whimpered to himself, battered, bruised and alone in bed at night, frightened to make a noise in case it brought another beating and further humiliation.

So what did Ben do? The only thing he could do. He escaped into his fantasy world, where he was big and strong and could beat his father into a pulp. He imagined himself huge, tough, impenetrable, invincible – and that is how he survived. At 13 he started body-building; his goal was to beat up his father. Had he felt the pain in the raw, on his own, he might not have survived. There certainly wasn't anyone there for him to tell.

Not surprisingly, as a young adult Ben became addicted to drugs, body-building and fantasy in the form of day-dreams, violent sci-fi films, and cultish/religious beliefs. He avoids reality as much as possible, wanting to be the centre of a world where he rules supreme. He can't trust people, especially women (who he feels have always let him down). His addictions help blot out the pain of the past. Yet, every time he has a relationship with someone, whether sexual or even friendship, up comes all of his suppressed rage, mistrust, grief and humiliation. Terrified of intimacy and what real closeness would cause him to face, he retreats back into his fantasy world, where life is simple, easy, and circulates round him. Real life is too dangerous to handle.

One of the reasons we can feel so reluctant to give up our addictions is precisely because they have been real allies in times of fear, loneliness and pain. And given the limited resources available to oppressed people, turning to addictions for help can seem to make good sense. After all, who else can you rely upon? Of course, the addictions have just served to hold the surface together to stop the bleeding; they have not cured the deep-down cause of the problem.

INDIVIDUAL RESPONSIBILITY

One of the problems with oppression is that it makes people feel powerless and hopeless. They can feel 'What's the point?' about virtually everything, especially about giving up addictions. 'Who cares if I'm hooked or not? I'm going to die anyway?' These attitudes arise from the accumulated distress of a lifetime's experience of being overpowered, ignored, brushed aside and abused. If you have always lost, it is hard to believe you will finally win. These negative attitudes are a major obstacle for oppressed people who want to get off the hook. It's almost as if you have to tackle powerlessness and hopelessness as a form of emotional addiction before you can get on to the main (or more obvious) addictions.

If you are oppressed, you may well feel like blaming someone for your situation. You might blame your family, or you might blame society. You might even blame yourself, thinking that if only you had been a better, stronger, more lovable and intelligent person, everything would have been different. This misplaced notion is usually the result of internalized oppression. In fact, the more powerless you feel, the more you usually want to find someone to blame.

But needing to blame actually keeps you powerless, and helpless. Of course, wrongs have been committed, and if you are a member of an oppressed group, your group has probably been dealt harsh blows. But continuing to act powerlessly will not change this situation. What you could do is to work towards changing society and its institutions as agents of oppression by participating in political action and campaigning for legal and social change. You can also overthrow the chains of your own oppression, once you've acknowledged that you have been oppressed.

It's Your Life

Being oppressed does *not* remove individual responsibility about getting hooked. To say, 'I've been oppressed as a young person and that is why I am a heroin addict,' might be true, but it is not the end of the story. It assumes you are powerless, that there is no such thing as the human will, the power of decision or individual intelligence. It is a negative belief that nothing can change, which is really only true as long as the painful emotions underlying the addiction remain unacknowledged and unreleased. You have the power to take responsibility for yourself and your life. Not to do that is to settle for far less than you deserve. It is your life, after all – and in Part Two of this book you can begin to take control of it in every aspect.

Part Two

Overcoming Addiction

Chapter 8

———■○■———

Making the Break

It is the 'Graveyard' session at a 'Giving Up Addictions Workshop': that is the first session after lunch, when people feel like curling up and snoozing, some even want to creep out, hoping nobody will notice. In the morning each person identified their main addiction and now they are going to look at 'making the break'. I have asked everyone to bring their 'props' with them – that is to say, the addiction that they are contemplating giving up.

OPEN COUNSELLING

Ray is divorced, aged 45, and a university lecturer. He has brought a bottle of vintage wine with him, because drinking alcohol, in particular good wine, is his main addiction. Before lunch, he 'owned up' that he drank too much, but couldn't face stopping. Ray has volunteered to be the subject of an open counselling session in front of the group, and he's laughing with embarrassment. The other people present have now perked up, eager to see what happens.

Ray and I stand in front of the group and I give him time to look around and get connected to people in the group. He is clearly embarrassed and I stay close to him, giving him encouragement and assuring him that he's safe. I explain that it's all right to feel and show any feeling that he needs to. He can say anything he wants. When Ray looks more comfortable I start the session.

CORINNE: 'So Ray, tell us, how often do you drink?'

RAY: *(pauses and looks embarrassed)* 'Every day, more at weekends.'

CORINNE: 'How much do you drink?'

RAY: *(pauses again)* 'Usually a bottle, sometimes two – once it's opened, I think, "it'll go to waste", so I drink it up. I seldom stop at one glass.'

CORINNE: 'Why do you drink?'

RAY: 'Well, it's a number of things, I sleep better after a few drinks, I get very wound up at work and need something to relax. And, I have to admit, I feel a bit lonely at night, especially at weekends, so it takes the edge off the loneliness.'

CORINNE: 'I see you brought this wine with you. . .'

RAY: 'Yes, it's my favourite. I love this wine.'

CORINNE: 'What do you love about it?'

RAY: *(laughs, embarrassed)* 'The taste is wonderful, it's warm and soothing; it dulls the edges. And, looking back, it reminds me of my dad, who used to drink the same wine. It was one of the few things we had in common.' *(Ray looks sad and pensive.)*

CORINNE: 'Why do you want to give it up if it means so much to you?'

RAY: *(looks down at floor)*, 'Well, I know I'm using it to shut off my feelings.'

CORINNE: 'Which feelings?'

RAY: 'Since my marriage broke up 3 years ago, I just haven't been able to trust any woman – again. *(Ray is on the edge of tears.)* But I'm beginning to want a relationship now and I realize that my drinking is holding me back.'

CORINNE: 'How?'

RAY: 'I guess it gives me an illusion of not being alone, so I don't actively seek company, especially late at night, when I feel bad.'

CORINNE: 'Why isn't that a good thing?'

RAY: 'Well, it's an illusion. In reality, I'm very lonely and I'm sick of it.'

At this point in the workshop I ask Ray to open his bottle of wine. He breathes in the aroma (laughing with embarrassment again), then he sighs. The wine clearly gives him lots of pleasure.

CORINNE: 'What would it be like to drink this right now, Ray?'
RAY: *(laughing)* 'Oooh, it would be lovely.' *(He starts to shake and sweat a little, his face flushing, his hands beginning to tremble as he gets in touch with his fear.)* 'I'd love it, mmmm.' *Ray laughs uncontrollably, letting out more fear and embarrassment.)*
CORINNE: 'Well, Ray, would you be willing to try something?'
RAY: 'Sure, anything.'
CORINNE: 'I'd like you to pour your wine down the sink, here.' *(pointing to the sink.)*
RAY: *(shocked)* 'What, you've got to be joking! Why?'
CORINNE: 'I'm asking you to do this because I think it will help you get in touch with your feelings. It's not a punishment and you don't *have* to do it if you don't want to.'
RAY: *(looks frightened, then sceptical, then laughs)* 'OK, I'll have a bash.'

What ensues is a counselling session, in which Ray pours his wine down the sink, drop by drop, while I ask him how he feels, what he's thinking, every inch of the way. The group has crowded round him and are giving him lots of encouragement and support. It is a very loving environment and Ray begins to sob like a baby as he pours the wine away. Many memories come back about 'good times' drinking with his dad, with his mates from school, at university, at work, but most of all, alone at home. By now, I am touching Ray's shoulders gently.

CORINNE: 'What would it be like to give this up for good?' *(Ray turns to me and hugs me, crying very hard.)*
RAY: 'I'll never be able to live without it, never. What am I going to do, it's all I've got?'

(He continues to cry hard for about 10 minutes. The whole workshop, including myself, is quiet, but beaming lots of heartfelt love and encouragement at Ray. One or two are wiping their own eyes, having been moved to tears of empathy by his show of emotions.)

CORINNE: *(gently)* 'Ray, I know you're hurting, keep on crying, don't stop, but try to take a look at the people around you.'

RAY: *(still crying, peeks out at the group and cries harder, hiding back in my shoulder.)* 'They must think I'm an idiot, behaving like this,' he cries.

CORINNE: 'No, Ray, we all think you're a very brave man. *(He cries even harder at this validation and the murmurs of agreement emanating from the group.)*

I continue working with Ray on releasing his isolation and fear until he's able to start connecting with group members. He begins to relax physically, although still trembling and sweating with fear.

CORINNE: 'What would you like to ask them, Ray?'

RAY: *(pauses, then says quietly)* 'Do you like me?'

Several members of the group put their hands up, and one by one they tell Ray what they like about him. As each person says 'I like your sense of humour', 'you're very warm and kind', or 'you're brave and honest', Ray laughs and cries a little, but is beginning to listen instead of shutting them out.

CORINNE: 'What would it be like to depend on people instead of wine?'

RAY: 'Oh, it would be wonderful. I can't imagine that anyone would want to help me, though.'

CORINNE: 'What would you need to do?'

RAY: *(thinks)* 'I guess I'd have to phone someone, especially at bedtime, but I feel I'd be a nuisance.'

I ask the group if anyone would be genuinely willing to let Ray phone them at bedtime for, say, 10 minutes. Three people put their hands up straight away. Ray is clearly touched by this offer, and cries again for a few minutes.

CORINNE: 'What would it mean to say goodbye to wine at bedtime?'
RAY: 'I'd be terrified, really scared of getting through the night. I'd feel so lonely and I might not sleep.'
CORINNE: 'What could you do about the loneliness?'
RAY: 'Well, I could phone these three at bedtime.' *(He laughs and looks shyly at the volunteers, still not believing their offers.)* 'If they really mean it.' *(All three nod enthusiastically. I have told people they should only offer what they believe they can stick to realistically.)* 'Well, that would be amazing.'

By now Ray is looking different – slightly flushed, relaxed, and much more approachable and human. He's been taking the first step towards 'making the break'. He's not forced to decide to give up on the spot, but he's been given a chance to *feel* what keeps him drinking – his unreleased grief about his father, his divorce, his isolation, low self-esteem and feeling unloved and unlovable. Seeing at least three people who want to 'be there' for him is a major contradiction to how he feels about himself. It gives him some breathing space, to test out for himself what it would be like not to drink at bedtime. At the end of this session (which took an hour), he decides to stop for a week and instead ring the three people who offered themselves to him as support.

A year later I had a letter from Ray, saying that this session was decisive in helping him give up alcohol. 'I looked into the jaws of my fear and saw it was just feelings, not reality. From that point I started reaching out to people and have done so ever since. That is not to say that there haven't been hard times, or relapses, but my isolation has begun to dissolve and I've recently started going out with a fellow lecturer – so something's definitely changed, and for the better.'

DECIDING WHAT YOU WANT

Getting rid of your addictions is not easy, but if you sincerely want to cut down or give up your addiction(s), it doesn't have to be that hard, either. What I have learned so far about 'making the break' (from my own experience and from counselling hundreds of people) is this:

- You alone can decide to do it; no-one else can do it for you.

- You will only do it when you WANT TO – when the benefits begin to outweigh the temporary 'feel good factor'.

- You may have attempted to give it up several times before and feel somewhat discouraged about trying again. DON'T BE. Very few people ever give up their addictions at the first attempt. It can take two, 10, or 20 attempts. No matter, you are going in the right direction each time you try.

- Sheer willpower isn't enough. It helps, but it isn't the whole story. You have to tackle the underlying chronic distresses.

- You must think about what you need in order to 'make the break' (as Ray did, above), and not do it in a self-punishing way that is bound to fail.

- You are not the only person in the world who is struggling with one or more addictions. Thousands, if not millions, are also trying to conquer similar problems.

- It is not your fault that you're addicted. You are not weak, unlovable, undeserving or 'bad'. You are on the 'Addictive Treadmill'.

- Only when you face and accept the reality of your addiction can you really start getting off the hook.

FACING AND ACCEPTING REALITY

Turn back your notebook to where you first listed your addictions in order of priority. Read them through again. Then decide which addiction you need to face right now, and write it down on a fresh page in your notebook. Immediately underneath, write down this 'first thought': what is scary about facing it?

....

....

Now that you have identified which addiction you want to cut down on or give up, and you know what scares you about facing this reality, try to accept that it is probably your fear of what will happen if you do cut down or give up that is keeping you hooked.

Accept reality: you are probably more scared of life without your addiction/s than with it/them because:

- You are scared of the discomfort of 'coming off'.

- You are frightened of being overwhelmed by feelings all the time.

- You fear that you won't be able to 'function' and go to work, run the house, have a social life, look after the children.

- You worry about being 'odd-one-out', explaining to your family, friends, workmates that you are going to change. You might fear their ridicule, being left out of social events, being thought 'weird'.

- You are anxious about being 'out of control' (this is especially scary if you are giving up tranquillizers/anti-depressants and/or sleeping pills, or have undergone treatment within the mental health system, as you can fear 'going mad').

If there is something else that scares you about life without your addiction(s), write it down in your notebook. Face up to it right there on the page.

....

....

HOW ARE YOU FEELING NOW?

By now you might be feeling very uncomfortable. Perhaps you have the urge to light a cigarette, make a coffee, turn on the TV, have a drink and/or throw this book out of the window. You might be cursing me for being a 'smart alec', or feeling extremely critical about what you are reading. This is a natural response to the fear that thinking about addictions nearly always brings up. You may be feeling very tired, or be distracted by something else you need to do. There might well be a battle going on between your chronic distress (which wants to keep you hooked on the Addictive Treadmill) and you (wanting to be in charge of your life). Remember: you are free to do exactly what you want. You do not have to go on reading if you don't want to, and you do not have to cut down or give up your addictions UNLESS YOU WANT TO.

Take a moment to ask yourself the following and note down your answers in your notebook:

Yes No

1. Would you like to like, even love, yourself?

2. Would you like to feel powerful and in control of your life?

3. Would you like to have better relationships?

4. Would you like to wake up and look forward to, rather than dread, the day?

Yes   No

5. Would you like to feel proud of yourself –
   including how you feel about your body?

6. Would you like to believe it when people say
   nice things to you about you?

7. Would you like to feel you are a better
   friend, partner, parent, colleague,
   employee?

8. Would you like to be able to handle criticism
   better?

9. Would you like to see your life progressing
   along the lines you want?

10. Would you like to stop repeating mistakes,
    and have a life that works positively in your
    favour?

11. Would you like to fulfil (or even just start
    naming) your wildest dreams?

If you have answered 'yes' to any of the above, then it seems
that you have accepted you are worth overcoming your
addictions. What you have to do now is to decide whether to
cut down or give up altogether. And to do that, you need to
prepare the ground.

PREPARING THE GROUND

The following steps are essential to your success in conquering
addictions. If you were a seedling, about to be planted out, you
would want to be given optimum conditions for your growth,

wouldn't you? So, give yourself the optimum conditions for growth as a human being. You deserve the very best.

Inform Yourself

Scour books, magazines, newspapers, TV and radio for information about your addiction. When your antennae become tuned, you will probably be amazed at the amount of information 'out there', waiting for you. The librarian at your local library will help you find relevant books, and might also have the address and phone number of a local self-help group. There are many voluntary organizations who offer free help and advice (such as the Eating Disorders Association if you think you're anorexic, bulimic or a compulsive eater or dieter). The Institute for the Study of Drug Dependency produces excellent booklets (for a small charge) on legal and illegal drugs. You need to become you're own expert. See the 'Help' section at the end of this book (pp. 275–88).

Talk to People to Get Support

One of the worst things about addiction is the silence and shame that surround it. Remember: we live in an addictive society, and it is 'normal' to be addicted to something. So really we are all in the same boat. You'd be surprised how many people are struggling in isolation with their everyday addictions. Find out about other people's experiences by being a good listener, and try to listen without judgement. It is probably easier to talk to close friends, family or your partner (if you have one) first. You might even talk to your employer or personnel officer (if you have one) if it is a caring company with a policy of helping with health problems. But do be selective about whom you talk to, and do not confide in gossips; protect yourself intelligently.

Find a Buddy

Getting off the hook is much easier if you don't do it completely alone. You may not feel like joining a group (either because you hate groups or haven't got the time), but you might find a buddy to cut down/give up with you. You can often find a buddy when you start talking to friends, work colleagues and family about your addiction. You can make a pact to do it together and have regular telephone and personal contact while you are giving up. You can agree to be confidential with each other, so you feel safe. You may even go to a group, a workshop or a conference on your particular addiction together, as it is often easier to go with another person than alone.

The best thing a buddy can do is to keep you to your cutting down/giving up deadlines and offer support if and when you crave. A buddy can also help you to measure your success and, overall, is the best antidote to isolation.

Get Professional Help

You might feel you need professional help with getting off the hook. Again, there are many agencies and voluntary organizations which offer free, confidential advice (see the 'Help' section). Or you might want to start with a visit to your General Practitioner, who might refer you on to addiction-specific professional help. Going to see a counsellor or a therapist might also help; again, you might be referred through your doctor, or you might want to contact someone directly (in which case you will have to pay, but will probably be seen much quicker). You can ask your GP to refer you on the NHS – but this may take time. If you can afford to go privately (fees vary), you can contact the British Psychological Society, the Women's Therapy Centre or ask in any local healing and natural health centres, and look at the 'Help' section at the back. Some voluntary organizations, like the Eating Disorders Association, have a register of local counsellors and you can always phone the Samaritans who could refer you on to a counsellor.

Join/Create a Support Group

Many people find support groups very helpful because they combat the isolation of feeling you are alone with your addiction and, more important, people can share their successes and failures. Immense support can be provided by a group of people in the same boat. It also can help take the heat off your family and friends who may be sympathetic, but can't really understand your problem as fellow survivors do.

A support group can also be invaluable if you live alone, or your family is hostile/unhelpful, and/or you have had a difficult time getting help through the established health service routes.

If you feel very strongly motivated, you might even set up your own support group (how to do this is covered in detail in Chapter 18: Positive Living).

MAKING THE DECISION

If you have faced and accepted reality about your addiction and you have started preparing the ground, then the decision as to whether you want to cut down or give up your addiction will probably be much less daunting. The decision may even form itself, without your having to do much at all.

Head and Heart, Working for You

Some people live in their heads, always letting their intellect and logic govern their lives. This can be very useful, because it means you are accustomed to preparing the ground, finding out all the facts you need and making an informed decision. The only danger when making a decision purely in your head, is that your heart and spirit might not want to follow it. You can make a 'head' decision not to eat cake and yet find yourself scoffing cream buns the minute you are near them, and then feel a terrible failure afterwards. This will almost inevitably be the outcome, if your head and heart are out of sync with each other.

There are also some people who live completely from their hearts, only ever doing what they 'feel like' and ignoring what their head says. Unfortunately, and equally predictably, you may be tricked by the 'feel good factor' into doing things which feel good, but harm you; and you might well be denying the truth of what you are doing to yourself because you do not want to face reality.

The best decisions are made by both the head and heart simultaneously. When your head and heart work in unison, you combine your best thinking with what's best for you on a feeling level – it is what some people call 'using your intuition'. If your head and heart become attuned to each other, you can lead your life in a more balanced way; you are not so split into 'I think I should give up, but I feel I don't want to'. Your head and heart tend to come together when you begin to heal emotionally, and this usually starts as you give up your addictions. You just have to learn to listen to your inner voice, which will get progressively easier to hear as you begin to thaw out.

Why You Need to Make a Decision

If you do not make a decision you remain powerless, and at the mercy of your chronic distress. Living in indecision can be agonizing. The worst situation of all is pushing it all to the back of your mind and hoping it will go away. It will not. The best part about making a decision is that *you're* in the driving seat, in charge of your life, moving forward. You might be frightened of making a decision about your addictions(s) because:

- You might make the wrong decision, which could be irreversible.

- You fear the unknown, and your addiction is at least habitual. You *know* what to expect.

- You don't know who you will be without it, so you feel insecure at the thought of giving it up (it feels like giving yourself up).

- You are worried that people won't like you any more.

- You fear not being able to stick with the decision, so you reason that it's better not to try, in case you disappoint yourself.

The Right Time is Now

Thinking there is a 'right time' to give up can lead you to procrastinate. You put off the evil day until you will 'feel more like it'. In fact, many of us feel we will finally decide to give up when things are less stressful. But life rolls on, or lurches on from crisis to crisis, and so the only right time is *right now*.

Life will always be stressful. However, that is *not* the same as saying things won't change or feel different – they will. And some changes will improve life. If you prepare the ground (especially by getting yourself positive support), you *can* give up your addictions.

CUT DOWN OR GIVE UP?

This is the big question everyone always asks, in the hope that 'cutting down' will be enough. It is not. There is really no short-cut to giving up, but giving up. Why?

- You can kid yourself that you have cut down when you have not really; you are simply continuing to deny that you're in trouble with your addiction.

- If you simply cut down, whenever pressure of daily life increases, your addictive behaviour will usually increase, too. If you know you start spending money like crazy before your menstrual cycle, and credit cards are a danger to you, then putting a spending limit on yourself probably will not work. Few people buy a bar of chocolate and eat only half of it. They buy it – and eat it all. Stopping half-way is very rare.

- Cutting down prevents the process of emotional healing that you need to work through. Only giving up completely will expose your distress, allowing it to surface and be released.

The Benefits of Giving Up

Fear can take over at this point. It can suddenly seem very unpalatable to be contemplating giving up your addiction now the crunch has come. So open up your notebook and remind yourself by writing down:

1. Why you want to give up.
   ....

2. What form of self-abuse you are tired of repeating.
   ....

3. Which personal benefits you hope will come from giving up.
   ....

4. What you are looking forward to about your new addiction-free life?
   ....

SETTING YOUR 'GIVING UP' DEADLINE

You can prepare the ground by informing yourself, talking to people, building your support and finding a buddy, but you still need to set your 'Giving Up' Deadline. If you have decided to give up your addiction, then look in your diary or at a calendar AND SET A REALISTIC DATE TO STOP.

1. Write it in your diary or on your calendar, and in your notebook NOW. How do you feel? Write down your reactions in the notebook. Yes, immediately under that important deadline!

   ....

2. Also write down a list of the people you are going to confide in and ask for their support.

   ....

   ....

Remember, you are doing this FOR YOU because you WANT TO – not because you HAVE TO.

Setting your 'Giving Up' date is a cause for celebration. Yes, you will feel scared of the stiff haul ahead without your addiction/s to 'help' you along. But many others have already taken that route and arrived safely. And they are all delighted that they did. Some got there just in time, before self-annihilation set in. Others feel it's a major brick in the edifice of their self-esteem and newly successful life.

Look at it this way. By deciding to 'make the break' you have decided:

- To put yourself first.

- To give up self-abuse.

- You are worth it.

- To live your life to the full.

- To fulfil your potential.

- To become fully human.

- To let your wildest dreams come true.

- To let the 'real you' emerge.

- To have fun.

- To end your isolation.

- To let yourself heal.

- Not to settle for less than absolutely everything.

- To give up basing your life on your frozen needs from the past, and meet your real needs in the present.

In other words, you have decided to be your own parent – a positive decision that will be fully discussed in Chapter 9.

Chapter 9

Being Your Own Parent

When you first give up an addiction, there is always that feeling that you have got to replace it with something. There is that empty hole, that yawning gap and you feel that you need to fill it – with an activity, a new habit, a person . . . something. Smokers know they reach for sweets and food, drinkers turn to cigarettes or soft or hot drinks – any drinks, compulsive TV watchers obsessively listen to the radio. Anyone giving up an addiction inevitably feels panicked by wondering what they're going to do instead. Suddenly there is extra time to fill. Social events don't seem so attractive, life seems bleak and boring, and/or you feel envious that others can indulge themselves with whatever they fancy, while you can't.

There is no substitute appropriate when giving up addictions other than going to the root of the problem and looking after yourself. I would be cheating you if I said: smokers should just chew special gum or drinkers should suck their thumbs, or compulsive spenders should just cut up their credit cards.

Such suggestions might deal with the immediate problem, but they do not, *cannot*, solve anything long-term, because the urges, the feelings beneath the addictive behaviours, are still there, lurking Jaws-like just under the surface. In fact, stopping the behaviour usually brings previously repressed feelings bubbling to the surface – so, initially, you can be in for a pretty rough time.

LEARNING TO LOVE YOURSELF COMPLETELY

Now for the *good* news: in my experience there is *one* substitute that does work long-term – AND THAT'S LEARNING TO LOVE YOURSELF COMPLETELY. You may think 'yuk' or 'impossible' at this point, but it really is the only permanent solution open to you. What is more, it is possible to learn to enjoy your life addiction-free – it can be a whole new way of being. Loving yourself brings immense rewards: such as being able to feel love from other adults, children, even animals.

Of course, you can try every type of 'cure' or 'therapy' going, and you may give up the habit short-term through hypnosis, drugs and/or willpower; but long-term, enjoyable, addiction-free life only comes when you love, forgive and nurture yourself *as if you were your own parent.*

Nurturing Yourself

Being your own parent means deciding to love and nourish yourself as if you were the most tender, precious and beautiful human being. I often ask clients how they would treat a delicate new-born baby, or a fragrant plant, or a much loved pet, and their eyes light up – the answer is obvious. They would lavish food, water, and tender loving care upon them. They would make sure that they were in the right temperature, and had a clean, comfortable environment. In other words, they would *nurture* them.

However, when I ask whether they would do the same for themselves there is usually a look of confusion, followed by embarrassed laughter and genuine wonder at such a ridiculous question. How selfish, how loathsome, how boring, what a waste of time, effort and money it would be.

Yet, this is precisely how we have to start, when we want to overcome our addiction. In Part One, we saw that we become addicted through a variety of experiences and pressures, such as pre-birth, birth itself, family life, school and further education/training, work and unemployment, relationships, crises and oppression. The root of addiction lies in *how* we have been hurt and whether we have been able to heal those hurts.

If the hurts are unreleased and instead accumulate, we end up with chronic distresses which can largely determine how we live our lives. The core of all addiction is isolation, self hatred, and unreleased pain (in particular our frozen needs). And if we carry this over into our teens, young adult, and adult life, even into old age, they limit our ability to treat ourselves (and others) well.

Learning to Connect

As we become inured to abuse and self-abuse, we think it's 'normal', 'natural', and 'how life is'. We also get used to being numb or to push down feelings once they start surfacing. As we saw in Chapter 2, we are very afraid of feeling our feelings, and addictions are a socially acceptable way of keeping us anaesthetized. Yet, we know now that on many psychological, emotional, physical, social and environmental levels, continuing to abuse ourselves leads eventually to self-destruction.

Healing can go on at many levels – and as you heal yourself from your inner, emotional hurts, so you will operate in your environment in a more respectful, loving and thoughtful way. If we are used to pouring toxins into ourselves, then we probably also pour toxins into those around us and our environment. But if we learn to nourish ourselves from the inside out, then we will find it harder to tolerate appalling social conditions and degrading inequality.

So deciding to nurture yourself isn't just a selfish, self-obsessed act. It is a step towards creating a better world, because you exist in that world, and you continue to create it (through your children, through work, through your actions).

Healing yourself necessarily has a positive, 'knock-on' effect for everything and everyone around you.

I have experienced this myself – as I have become more connected to myself, have treated myself better, nurtured my health through alternative health therapies and swimming; learned to eat better, learned to rest; worked on my inner life through counselling, therapy and meditation, and allowed my artistic self to be expressed through singing, dancing, acting, writing, and so on. I have made new friends with positive outlooks. I have attracted many new counselling clients and journalistic work to me. I have even welcomed a cat into my life – and I have always been allergic to them until now.

It is as if my healing of myself through a variety of means has made me more attractive, open, fun to be with. I am more alive; I have a better memory; I am more trustworthy and reliable. I have become more tender (my plants even get watered regularly and effortlessly), and I now feel easy spending time with myself – just being, and enjoying being, me.

But this is not a life devoid of deep feeling. It is a life filled with the whole gamut of human emotions – from joy to sorrow. I've probably cried more in the last year than in the previous five years, but it has done me a lot of good. I have felt depths of dark despair, grief and fear, and I have lived through them with a lot of help from my friends. My isolation has been thawing. I feel more intense love, compassion and connection for other human beings, for animals and for the world, as I feel myself to be part of the universe.

Giving Up Waiting

The most important decision of all has been to give up waiting. I have waited all these years to find my long-lost twin, the perfect partner, the most romantic and sexy lover, the ideal job, the most wonderful therapy, the most gorgeous baby – and I have begun to realize they simply don't exist. Real life is messy, unsorted out, and some things are unresolvable. I always wanted to be perfect – and now I know I am not. What a relief; I am human after all. I can partake of things human, such as intimacy, closeness, pain and pleasure. I am enough for myself, complete and separate, and I can take whatever time I need to get where I want to go.

Yet many people are still waiting – for the right person to come along, for the mega pools or premium bond win, for that call to Hollywood, for the day the scales finally indicate a loss of two stone in weight, for an apology from someone who hurt them. And they are waiting in vain. The trick to living life to the full is to give up waiting. *Nobody – absolutely nobody – but you is in charge of your life.* You, and only you, can make your life what you want it to be and the time to start is right now. So stop waiting.

- You will never, ever have the perfect parents and family you always wanted.

- You will never, ever be able to change your body size, hair colour, facial features, height, and so on to fully satisfy your idealized image of how you should be. There will always be something else that you judge to be not quite right.

- You will never, ever be able to eradicate your class background, your ethnic/racial heritage, your skin colour – no matter how hard you try. It is rather something to celebrate and be proud of anyway.

- You will never, ever be able to tailor your sexuality to fit society's exacting prescriptions.

- You will never, ever be clever, intelligent, witty enough to beat everyone else at *Brain of Britain* or *Mastermind*.

- You will never, ever be able to change one second of your past. It is over, it happened (all those horrendous things as well as all those brilliant things).

Living in the Present

The only thing to do RIGHT NOW is to recognize that you are living in the present. Each second of life is a fresh second, never experienced before, and so fleeting it can never be experienced again. Certainly, the past is determined – it is past. It is over. But the future is undetermined and as you are reading this you can choose to do anything you want with this present moment. You can carry on reading or do something else – it is up to you. And what you do next is also up to you. That you have always done something this way or that way . . . is history. You can do something different . . . RIGHT NOW. You can CHOOSE.

And this is also true of your addictions. You might well have been on the Addictive Treadmill: drinking yourself silly, smoking 40 cigarettes a day; masturbating over porn every night; starving yourself; over-spending on credit cards every day – that is, up until this moment. I suggest your starting point is learning to be your own parent: to nourish, love, care, forgive yourself, and start again. This minute.

Of course, the desire to fill your frozen needs (all those needs in the past that were not met), is the driving force behind the Addictive Treadmill. But you can throw the switch and stop the machine – you can step off right now. You can decide to step off any time you like. You are not welded to it forever.

Building Your Self-Esteem

Along with deciding to step off the Addictive Treadmill, you need to build your self-esteem. Only you can do this. No matter how many times people tell you they like you, love you, adore the colour of your eyes, think you are clever, admire you – it will not make any real difference until you are ready to take it into yourself and use it positively.

If you want to live an addiction-free life, then build your self-esteem. Addictions have got nothing to hang on to when you like yourself. They leech you dry when you loathe yourself, but they slide right off you when you think you're great. Why would you want to hurt someone so nice with harmful addictions? Why would you want to abuse someone so beautiful?

MEETING YOUR REAL NEEDS

The remaining chapters in Part Two of this book are designed to help you to identify your real needs and to start meeting them for yourself. Of course, there is a lot of overlap between all of these needs – but they have been separated out for clarity. They are:

- Emotional Needs

- Physical Needs

- Sexual Needs

- Social Needs

- Creative Needs

- Intellectual Needs

- Spiritual Needs

Seeing them all listed like that can seem pretty daunting. BUT be easy on yourself – remember:

- You do not have to deal with them all at once. Take it step by step; perhaps start with the area you feel you have some chance of changing.

- You do not have to adhere to every suggestion rigidly (or kick it all out as impossible either). Dip into a chapter that attracts you and try just one or two things (we can get very rigid when we give up addictions).

- You are doing this for you and nobody else.

- It will take time to change. You might be feeling desperate, impatient, and frustrated – but changing takes time, effort, determination and persistence. Give yourself the time you need.

- You may not succeed straight away; you may have several false starts. Keep reminding yourself that you are going in the right direction.

- Try to enlist support, encouragement, help. You don't have to do it in splendid isolation (even though it's up to *you* to do it). It is not cheating, to depend on people who are dependable. It is an intelligent, and positive strategy.

- The past is over. You are now taking on board a whole new way of looking at your life. Give up the addiction, and instead fill yourself and your life with all the good things you really need.

- You are making a positive commitment to yourself.

- This way lies power, self-fulfilment, and happiness.

Chapter 10

—◉—

Meeting Your Emotional Needs

We all have emotions; that is what makes us human. Yet, owning up to being 'emotional' and having 'emotional needs' can be difficult, because as we have already seen in Chapter 2, being open and vulnerable can make you feel that you are 'weak'. And, as you have also learned, the purpose of addiction is to suppress and distort your emotions. So, when you decide to get off the hook, you usually start experiencing a wide range of feelings as you begin to thaw.

POWERFUL 'MEDICINE'

You might feel scared that you're getting 'out of control' because you feel weepy, irritable, exhausted, flat, confused and/or afraid. But you can learn to handle your emotions, if you want to. The flip side is that you begin to feel more alive, less tied to the Addictive Treadmill, less frightened of feeling real feelings and actually more in control. So deciding to meet your own emotional needs by getting wise about them and being clear about what you want, is the single most powerful thing you can do to help yourself stay off for good.

It is important to remember that:

- It is completely 'normal' and 'healthy' to have emotional needs.

- Profound emotional healing can take place 'naturally', if we allow ourselves to release our hurts fully.

- Physical health is very closely connected to our emotional health. The more we suppress our feelings, usually the worse our health will be (especially long-term).

- Focusing on positive emotions (love, joy, happiness, affection), creates positive energy which in turn triggers a positive force in your life.

- Men and women are equally emotional. The apparent difference is because women are encouraged to show some emotions, such as grief and fear, and suppress others, such as anger, while men are encouraged to do the reverse.

- Having emotional needs is nothing to be ashamed of.

- Feelings are feelings – nothing more, nothing less.

- Neither 'good' nor 'bad' emotions are to be feared. They are to be acknowledged, accepted, welcomed, revelled (not wallowed) in, and enjoyed to the full.

- Becoming 'emotionally literate' means understanding your emotions, and other people's emotions, so you can act powerfully in your life.

FROZEN NEEDS

As we also saw in Chapter 2, much of life can be spent futilely trying to meet frozen needs: those real needs which were not met adequately (or at all) when we needed them to be met in the past.

What Are Your Frozen Needs?

Open up your notebook again and jot down your answers to the following questions.

1. What do you long for? Crave? Feel hopelessly attached to?

   ....

2. Do you need endless praise and lots of reassurance?

   ....

3. Do you want people to tell you that you are lovable, irresistible, brilliant?

   ....

4. Do you feel you would love to be famous?

   ....

5. Do you feel a yawning, empty gap inside that you long to fill?

   ....

6. Are you looking for a mum and/or a dad, a family or sisters and brothers, and/or ex-lovers in your current relationships?

   ....

7. Do you feel 'if only' a lot of the time?

   ....

8. Do you feel no matter how much love/money/sex/attention/work you have it will never be enough?

   ....

9. Do you seldom feel really satisfied – that you want more and more and more?

   ....

10. Do you often feel hungry and thirsty, even though you have just eaten and drunk?

....

If any of these questions evoked a 'yes' response from you, then you've definitely got frozen needs.

11. Can you be more specific about what you know about your own frozen needs? Remember, no-one but you need ever see this notebook. Don't cheat on yourself at this stage in your recovery programme. Write down exactly what it is that you feel your frozen needs are.

....

Giving Up Frozen Needs

Now that you have honestly assessed your frozen needs, there's only one thing to do with them – and that is to give them up. Forever. Otherwise, they will lead you back to the Addictive Treadmill. Decide, RIGHT NOW, to give them up for good. In 'being your own parent', you have to look after yourself, so it is important to give up waiting for someone else to do it for you. Giving up your frozen needs is a big leap towards overcoming addiction.

Holding a Direction

To help yourself to do this, it is useful to say out loud to yourself a few words of positive direction for change (otherwise known as a 'direction' or 'affirmation').

You might feel silly, shy or bored at the very idea, but saying a 'direction' speaks straight to your subconscious, to the 'inner you', and can bring about profound changes in your attitude to life, if you repeat it to yourself several times a day. As you say a 'direction' you may find yourself shaking, yawning, crying, laughing, feeling self-conscious, lethargic or any mixture of these.

Try saying the following 'direction' to yourself in a positive tone while sitting or standing comfortably, and/or looking in a mirror. Complete the sentence by saying the 'first thought' that pops up in your mind (this will tell you what you really know/feel subconsciously):

'I cheerfully promise, from this moment on, I will stop trying to fill my frozen needs for (love, sex, fame, food, praise, a mother, a father, money, being perfect — include whatever makes sense to you), and instead I decide right now to meet my real needs for myself. This means
....
....

Try saying this ten times over and see what comes to mind as you go (it's a good idea to note down both the 'direction' and your responses). Say this direction in the morning, when you're in the bathroom, and/or at lunchtime, if you have 10 minutes alone, and/or at bedtime, before you go to sleep.

Once you've begun to identify your real needs (for instance, for a mutual, loving friendship, a well-paid job in a pleasant environment or an hour of solitude every day), you are on track for meeting those needs.

Assessing Your Real Needs

Take a moment now to think about your 'real needs'. What are they? Study the following categories, one to six, and then write down in your notebook all the relevant needs you come up with.

1. For yourself, generally?
....

2. At work?
....

3. At home?
....

4. In love relationships?
....

5. In friendships?

....

6. With your children (if you have them)?

....

BUILDING YOUR SELF-ESTEEM

Building your self-esteem is not the same as being 'big-headed', a 'show-off', or an 'arrogant bore'. Learning to love yourself for who you are is central to giving up addictions, because if you no longer hate, loathe or punish yourself for being 'bad', then self-abuse becomes completely unappealing.

How to Build Your Self-Esteem:

Here is another exercise to complete in your notebook, as and when appropriate – some suggestions do not involve note-making.

1. List 20 things you like about yourself. Add five more qualities to this list each day. Keep the list with you, and remind yourself of them by reading them through at least once a day. More often if you are feeling a bit low.

2. Every time you do anything, think of three things you are pleased about in terms of how you have done it. For instance, if you have decorated a room, tell yourself what it is *you* like about your colour choice, handiwork, etcetera, and congratulate yourself on your achievement (*especially* if it's not perfect).

3. Ask people for positive feedback (we are all very bad at this). Be pro-active in asking your family, 'What do you love about me?', or your friends, 'What do you like about me?' or your partner, 'What do you most love about me?/ what is good about being with me?' Ask your boss, 'What did you like about the [tasks] I've just completed?' and,

'What do you think is most commendable about the way I do my job?' Be prepared to prompt people to say positive, rather than negative things, because we are all so used to being criticized rather than praised. You may feel very awkward at first, being so direct with people, but it will tell you more about yourself. Note down what people say and when you get home, transfer their comments to your notebook. Then read over these comments next time you see them or approach a task.

4. Remember your successes, and build on them. It's very easy to put yourself down at every opportunity for being a failure, not being high enough up the career ladder, never having done anything 'special' with your life. Think back to the exams you have passed, skills you have acquired, people you have got close to and loved (and who have loved you). Write them down in your notebook. Also note moments you're proud of, such as doing first aid on an injured person after an accident; babysitting for a friend who needed to get out of the house; letters and poems you have written; meals you've cooked and/or any number of other things. Especially note down things you have done that went against your fear: for instance, perhaps you were frightened of water and learned to swim in your twenties? Maybe you are terrified of busy main roads, but passed your driving test anyway?

5. Forgive your mistakes. We can be so hard on ourselves about mistakes we make. And we do all make them. Yet, it is easy to slide into negativity if you feel that you are a 'bad person' and you've messed things up. The best thing to do if you have made a mistake is own up to it. Don't pretend you haven't done it when you have. Face the fact that you made a mistake and make adequate amends; don't blame someone else – that is powerlessness breaking through. Equally, don't go 'over the top' by over-compensating). If you have broken someone's vase, say, 'I'm very sorry' (and mean it) and replace the vase – but not with one that is far more expensive or much cheaper. If you have forgotten to

post a letter to someone, don't lie or pretend; own up and rectify the situation.

6. Stop trying to be perfect: it's impossible. Be 'good enough', instead. Low self-esteem can drive you to need to be perfect, impeccable, spotless, unreproachable. This can make you fastidious, over-meticulous, a procrastinator, and very hard on yourself because you are not 'perfect'. Human perfection is an illusion. Yes, you should strive for the best for yourself (and others), but no-one can be the perfect husband, parent, child, friend, or employee. At some point you will forget something important at work or say something mean to a friend – to err is human. Giving up perfectionism goes hand in hand with forgiving yourself. If you do both simultaneously, you will have more breathing space to explore being perfectly imperfect.

7. Learn to Love Your Body. Take off your clothes and look at yourself in a long mirror for five to 10 minutes. Feel your skin, look at its textures. Admire your curves and muscles. Look closely at your eyes and face; enjoy yourself. Notice your shape, size, height, the different colours of hair on your body. Look at the shape of your hands and feet, the curves of your legs and arms. Don't stand there wishing you were different, accept who you are, just as you are – you are fine. Write down in your notebook the things you like about your body: your hair, eyes, mouth, hands, legs, buttocks, and so on.

8. Act as if you are a success, you are well-loved, you like yourself. Building your self-esteem is all about loving and accepting yourself, while acting powerfully. Most of us don't realize even a third of our potential in life. If you want to make your dreams come true, you will have to plunge in and start somewhere. For example, if you want to be popular, you will not achieve it sitting at home, waiting for someone to ring, feeling self-pity because you have not been asked out. Ask someone out to the cinema; invite people round to eat with you – it doesn't have to be an elaborate meal or event.

Act as if you are a successful, interesting person, and you will be moving towards becoming one. But don't pretend – 'acting as if' is not based on pretence. It is about challenging your fears and stepping further out into your life. Once you start, you will feel better about yourself, because you will be making evident progress.

9. Treat yourself well. Your self-esteem simply won't grow if you always treat yourself badly. (The rest of Part 2 of this book is all about this, especially Chapter 11, which is about meeting your physical needs (health, fitness, diet, exercise, etc.) If you treat yourself well, you will feel better about yourself, you'll look better, you will treat others better, which will improve your relationships, which in turn will increase your self-esteem. (This is especially important if you have children – or are thinking of having them – because they will model themselves on you.)

10. Notice who loves/likes you. In your notebook, make a list of all the people who love you (and whose love you can feel and accept). Make another list of people who like you. You may feel very unsure of whether people like or love you, or not, so practise remembering what they say or do with you, how you feel when you are together, what you notice about their enjoyment at being with you. Assume people will like you, because if you expect a negative outcome, you will probably get one. Whereas, if you expect to be liked, that communicates itself in your demeanour, and it will be very attractive. When someone compliments you, accept it gracefully, say 'thank you', don't reject it. Learn to take, learn to trust.

11. Learn to say 'no'. We often feel we must instantly agree to do something when asked, largely because we fear other peoples' anger or disapproval, or because we believe we are only 'good' if we appease and please. Try saying, very lightly, 'Thanks for asking me, but I'm sorry I won't be able to accept/do x or y, etc.' If you are not sure whether you want to say 'yes' or 'no', buy yourself some time. Say 'I would like to think about it and get back to you tomorrow.'

If you are pressurized to make a decision on the spot, and you really don't want to, then don't.

12. Be assertive, not aggressive. When you first start building your self-esteem and you have been shy, or a doormat, or timid, there can be a tendency to go to the other extreme and be aggressive about everything. A more balanced approach is to be assertive, not aggressive. Be firm, be pleasant, be light, but say straight out what you want. 'No thank you, I don't want a cigarette/drink/second helping', said with a smile, communicates that you don't want what is being offered, but you are not rejecting the offerer. A good example is when people come round selling anything from religion to clothes pegs on your doorstep. If you don't want to buy, open the door, smile, but say very firmly, 'No thank you. Goodbye', and close the door again, before they get their foot and sales patter in. You have been firm, clear, but not rude.

13. Put Yourself First. Expect to get what you need, ask for it and notice when you get it. This does not mean being selfish, egocentric, greedy and grabbing. It means being clear about your needs, being straight with yourself and others about what you do and do not want, taking time to feel/think about what does you good. If you put yourself first, consciously, then you will enable people around you to put themselves first, too. Just believe that you are worth it.

RELEASING YOUR EMOTIONS

Profound emotional healing can take place when your emotions are faced and released. So, if you want to give up your addictions, learning to release your emotions is essential. You can become very 'tuned in' to your feelings and cease to be scared of, or thrown by them. At root there are three 'core' emotions: anger, grief, and fear. Other emotions, such as jealousy, envy, humiliation and resentment, stem from these three, often being a complex mixture.

Listening to Your Inner Voice

If you sit quietly for a few minutes and 'tune in' to how you are feeling by asking yourself, 'How am I feeling, right now?' your 'inner voice' might answer back both as a feeling from your solar plexus (centrally under your ribs), and an actual voice in your head. Close your eyes and just notice how you are feeling right now: on edge? tired? happy? bored? don't really know? numb? fed up? a bit weepy? OK?

It is important to keep asking yourself, as you move through the day, how you are feeling. Notice how your moods change, what lifts you 'up', what pushes you 'down'. Notice how you feel with different people. Notice how you feel before doing a task: you have got to do the washing up – how do you feel? You are off out dancing with friends – how do you feel? Your children are home from school demanding attention and food – how do you feel? Are there particular times during the day when you feel most 'together'? Are there times when you regularly feel rather down?

Your inner voice is the 'me' that talks back to you quietly inside. If you have a habit of talking to yourself (many sane people do), then you will already be talking to the inner you. If you have small children, pets or plants, you might talk to them as an indirect way of talking to yourself. Get used to noticing how you really feel. It might well be the whole gamut of feelings. Don't try to repress the 'bad' emotions you think are 'unacceptable', such as jealousy, envy, hatred. Just accept that you can feel a wide range of feelings at any one moment.

Listening to Your Head and Heart

Your inner voice is a reliable indication of what you are really feeling. Some people operate from thinking more than feeling, saying things like, 'I *should* visit the dentist', or 'I *ought* to help my parents move house'. Of course, knowing what you think is essential for coping with life's complexities. But if we always live by our 'oughts' and 'shoulds', we are really living by duty and obligation, rather than doing what really makes sense for ourselves.

It can be quite difficult to disentangle what you think you 'should' do and what you 'feel like' or 'want' to do. Many of us are so tied up with principles and beliefs which give us rules for living, that we often do precisely the opposite of what we want to do, purely because we 'ought'. Yet actions which come out of a sense of duty are not necessarily the best actions, because your heart isn't in them – and it very often shows. You might be half-hearted in helping someone because you don't really want to, but think you 'should'. However, if you are beginning to live your life according to your own, rather than other peoples' rules, in order to overcome your addictions, then you might have to allow yourself to do things out of passion, conviction and/or genuine desire, rather than out of a rigid strait-jacket of duty.

As with everything, you need to find a balance, and it might take some time to 'tune in' to your real desires, if you have never done it before. If you have always been told what to do, you might feel that you 'don't know' what you want/feel or think at any given moment. Don't panic. In time, with practice and emotional healing, it should get easier. You don't have to force it. Be patient with yourself. Just learn to listen to how you really feel every day. It will gradually become 'second nature' to you.

When you can listen to your head and your heart, and both seem to be working together, then you will be operating in a much more balanced way. It may seem scary at first to trust to your 'intuition' (which is really a balanced mixture of your head and heart when they're working well together), but in time you will just 'sense' what's right for you. Trust your instinct.

LOSING CONTROL TO FIND YOURSELF

Because most of us have been brought up to 'control' our feelings, be polite, count to ten when angry, and so on, what I am now going to tell you might seem strange. It may take you some time to lose control, but the benefits can be enormous. Instead of living your life carrying barrel-loads of pent-up feelings, you can learn to face, accept *and* release your emotions, which will further free you from the Addictive Treadmill.

If you have ever watched children express their emotions, you will have noticed that they can cry very hard, scream and rage, and then, almost immediately, switch their attention to playing or looking at something interesting, or interacting with other children, once they have unleashed the upset. If you want to release your feelings in order to get off the hook permanently, then you'll have to 'relearn' how to act like a child. This is *not* to say that you should throw tantrums in stores or scream at your boss, or attack your family with a meat-cleaver, but you need to recognize the fact that you have your emotional equipment for a reason, and if you can allow it to work naturally, then you can heal your past (and current) hurts.

Of course, you can't simply let rip wherever and whenever you want, that would be neither appropriate or effective. In fact, it could be counter-productive, seriously jeopardising your job, or your social life. But you can learn what you need in order to lose control and then set things up in your life so you can access this form of release regularly.

At the same time you might think you're 'not the kind of person' to show your feelings. You might feel shy, inhibited or frightened of what might come out. But if you are a human being, then you are by definition 'the kind of person' who has emotions, and you may surprise yourself by actually enjoying the act of unleashing them, because you will almost certainly feel more alive.

Get Wise About Letting Go

Here are some of the ways in which you can let go of your feelings. It is important for you to understand how your own emotions work because everyone's are different. Some of the following could work for you, or you might prefer to develop your own ways of releasing feelings. Whatever you decide, give yourself licence to feel and experiment. After all, you are in charge.

Telling the story.   If you need to let go of an 'upset' or more serious incident, such as a car crash or the end of an intimate relationship, you will need to talk about it. You will need to find a sympathetic ear, someone who will really listen and not interrupt your flow. And you will need to 'tell the story' over and over, and over, from beginning to end. As you tell the story you will probably experience other feelings, such as anger, grief, and fear. If you are telling the story while feeling numb and flat, then you will need to go back to the beginning again and let yourself stay more in touch with your real feelings.

If you can't think of anyone to talk to, then talk into a cassette recorder (and record yourself). But don't play back the tape for at least a month, and *never* send it to anyone to 'prove' how upset you are. You can also sit and talk to a teddy bear, pet budgie, cat, dog, and/or a favourite tree or a star.

Of course, you may find a good friend (or several) and/or your partner or family might listen while you tell the story, but you will need to talk about the incident a great deal and sometimes family and friends can begin to feel that you are 'too demanding'. Don't take it too personally. It is just that other people have their own needs and sometimes can't listen. We often have unrealistic fantasies that we can be 'saved' by one particular person. But no one person has enough 're-sources', so you will need to tap many to meet your need to be listened to. If you feel that none of the 'listeners' suggested above can meet your needs, do consider phoning the Samaritans, who provide an excellent 24-hour listening service, and/or professional counselling/therapy.

Writing. This is similar to telling the story. Some people find it a great relief to 'get it out of their system' by writing a letter and/or writing in a diary where they 'say everything', when they are feeling hurt. It is *not* a good idea to post any letters you write at such times, because in a letter written out of deep, gut-level pain, you will say many things you will probably regret. You will lose your dignity – by attacking, grovelling, accusing, ranting at, blaming someone who you feel has hurt you. So, when you have poured out your emotions, put the letter/s away in a drawer and let it/them remain there for a week or so. Later, when you've recovered from the immediate pain, and read through what you wrote, you will probably be relieved you didn't send it. But writing impassioned, uncensored letters and/or a journal can bring immense relief. Some people even turn their pain into fiction, drama, non-fiction articles and books. This is a good idea, but bear in mind that any self-revelation may come back and hit you, boomerang-style, even if it is heavily disguised. Be prepared for the possible consequences.

Grief. This is obviously released through crying. However, there are different kinds and intensities of crying available to us. Mostly people do their utmost to repress their tears in polite society, dabbing at their eyes to stem the flow and sniffing into their handkerchief, because having a good howl is 'socially unacceptable'. Men especially find it hard to 'let go', because they have been conditioned to be tough and 'manly' (although this is changing). Delicate eye-dabbing might well be appropriate on the bus to work, or in the bank queue, but you will definitely benefit from having a really good, gut-shaking howl as soon as possible. This may cause discomfort, rather like cramps in the solar plexus, but will also bring immense relief through healing. You can get a good howl by taking yourself off to a place where it doesn't matter if you cry – like alone in a wood, or by the sea, when nobody's around. But best of all, is to be at home listening to a piece of heart-rending music, and/or watching a sad film, reading a sentimental poem or anything else that 'triggers' off your tears. Let them flow until they cease naturally.

If you are bereaved and feel you need to cry, but can't get to the feelings very easily, it is a good idea to deliberately trigger yourself off by looking at favourite photos, fondling clothes, smelling perfume/aftershave, remembering the 'good times' you had together, going back to special places, re-reading letters, talking to mutual friends about what you loved about the person. Any or all of these strategies will usually make your grief more accessible.

Don't forget that grief goes through many stages – of numbness, depression, feeling 'fed up', heavy, weepy, before you can get to actual crying. Learn to recognize how you feel just before you break into tears. Is it a lump in the throat? A pricking behind the eyes? A tightening in the chest and solar plexus? Whatever the warning signs, just allow the feelings to well up and brim over. It may help you to howl deeply if you hold a cushion very close to your solar plexus. Best of all, would be to hug someone extremely close to you, and/or have someone put their arms round you and simply let you cry.

Most of us try to 'shush' someone when they cry, or try to distract them, because we feel awkward about their tears. If your companion tries to do either of these things just say, 'It's fine, don't worry. I know what I need to do. Just hold me close'. If the other person clearly finds this difficult, it might be safer for you if he or she goes away and leaves you to grieve alone. Simply do whatever makes it safe for you to cry. You might also find it helps to get into bed and snuggle under your duvet or steep in a warm bath. Once you feel secure, the grief should well up automatically.

Other people can get very worried by overt shows of strong emotion, like grief, and may need to be reassured that you are not 'cracking up'. There is so much fear about showing emotions in public that it is inevitable that you will find some weird reactions to you releasing your feelings. But if you stick to what you know you need (and everyone sees that you are absolutely fine afterwards), then they will get used to your being in touch with yourself.

After a 'good cry' you will probably feel emotionally lighter, relaxed and relieved. Indeed, the chemical content of tears cried in grief are different from tears cried while cutting onions. Natural tranquillizers, called endorphins, are released into the blood stream when you grieve, creating a feeling of calm after the storm. Another plus factor is that if you get used to grieving (and your friends, family and colleagues get used to it, too) you make it easier for them to show their feelings to you. Don't allow anyone to put you down, or ridicule you for being a 'cry baby'; it's just their discomfort talking.

Anger/rage. Most of us are frightened of our anger. Of course, when anger gets out of hand it can be accompanied by violence, which can terrify, injure, even kill. Many of us carry frightening memories of adults being angry with us as children or being bullied by peers (or older children) at school and at home, so we can feel very small, vulnerable and helpless when people are angry.

If you have a 'bad temper' or 'fly off the handle' inappropriately, you may need to learn to control it when it is detrimental to you to show it (and/or where you may inflict harm on somebody by hitting out). Instead, it is best to find an appropriate outlet either on your own or with someone else who can ride the storm so you can release your anger safely.

A couple of tried and tested means of releasing anger (in private) are:

- Loud talking or shouting – where you say things like 'you bastard', 'how dare you' or, 'go away', or whatever you need to say about what has made you angry. This can feel unreal or awkward, and indeed some people 'dramatize' their anger this way. However, it can lead to the release of real fury, which is usually white hot and unmistakable, accompanied by sweating, blushing and/or shaking.

- Making violent movements – bashing cushions, kicking things, throwing things (try soft balls against a brick wall or hitting the wall with a pillow, as in a pillow fight), this can be accompanied by a loud shout or growling, deep from your solar plexus. To ensure the least disturbance for your neighbours and family, it is a good idea to shout into a pillow or cushion, or best of all, go out into an open space where no-one can hear.

A very good place to shout is in a car (if you have one). But don't use your car as a battering ram as some people do in road rage attacks – it's far safer to shout in the privacy of your own vehicle. You can also stand under a railway bridge and shout as the train passes over, or shout facing out to sea, or go to a football match or other sporting event and shout at the opposing team. (You might instead play a hard and fast game, like squash, badminton or swim twenty lengths of the pool at high speed.) You can also shout at the TV if things are annoying you, but make sure that you don't frighten other people in your household, or neighbourhood – it's best to do it when alone or with someone who understands.

Don't shout or rage at people who don't deserve to be shouted at, even though the temptation may be to 'have a go' at someone. We tend to victimize other people when we feel victimized and, unfortunately, there is usually a pecking order. For example, a boss shouts at a man, the man shouts at his wife, his wife shouts at their child, who punches a smaller child and kicks the dog, which makes the smaller child punch even smaller children while the dog chases a cat, who then tyrannizes a mouse, and so on.

If you need to stand your ground with someone who's shouting at you, then shouting back may well shut them up, especially if you are usually quiet and accommodating. But on the whole it is a good idea to get your anger out as and when you first feel it building. But *don't* direct it at any one in particular. Also, don't take your anger out on yourself through self-mutilation or other addictive abuse. Sometimes we do this as a way of breaking through the numbness, so we can get to the feelings lurking underneath. Just remember: if you can tune in to your anger *before* you hurt yourself (or anyone else) either physically or emotionally, you will be in charge of your anger rather than it being in charge of you. Eventually, this will become second nature to you.

Fear. There are many ways to release fear, some of which we already practise automatically. Fear manifests itself as cold and hot sweats; clammy hands; uncontrollable shivers and trem-bles – knees knocking, teeth chattering; embarrassed laugh-ter, such as giggling; raucous laughter, such as hysterics, or belly-laughing that might be stimulated by watching a good comedian, funny film or joking at work; numbness, blankness and feeling 'frozen', which makes you unable to move, feel or think.

You can release fear deliberately before, during and after experiencing something scary. It is a particularly good idea to release it *before* something important in your life, such as a job interview, getting married, making a speech or having a driving test, because it will enable you to function efficiently during the event itself. Often people get a 'delayed reaction', shaking uncontrollably after something shocking such as an accident, or tragic news.

If *you* are worried about showing fear during an important public event, you will probably notice prior to the event that you are getting a dry mouth, a desire to giggle uncontrollably at the slightest thing, a feeling of clammy hands, a lump in the throat or 'butterflies in the stomach'. You can make yourself release fear quite deliberately, by allowing yourself to shiver and laugh while contemplating all the things that could possi-bly go wrong on the day. (Try 'shimmying' your shoulders to get the shakes started.)

It is also a good idea to watch funny programmes, flick through a favourite joke or cartoon book, or remember some jokes, to make yourself laugh. Laughter is *the* antidote to fear. It is also profoundly physically healing. You can also go to fun-fairs, horror movies, read thrillers and use other 'scary' expe-riences to release fear. The unbridled screaming that goes on on the ghost train or big dipper is extremely useful – it is only unproductive when you are so genuinely scared that you clam up altogether.

Fear can be ridden, like surfing on a huge wave. It can actually be exhilarating and exciting – in fact, this is how people who love danger can turn fear from something menac-ing into something alluring (but they also have to take care that they don't become addicted to the adrenalin-thrill of fear). If you can imagine yourself riding a wave instead of being swept away by fear, you can harness it to help you live the life you want.

People also fear fear. Panic attacks are really just huge globs of fear trying to get out of your system very quickly. People are often taught to breath to control panic attacks, but I tend to think this merely suppresses the fear and does not 'cure' the panic. Panic attacks usually occur when you are in a situation which reminds you of earlier or similar ones that were frightening. Because we tend to panic about the panic, we feel we are going to be swamped by terror. So we panic at the natural symptoms of fear, such as a racing heart, difficulty in breathing or wanting to escape.

You will only get long-term relief from this fear if you can learn to release the feelings which created the panic in the first place. You will probably need to shake, shiver, laugh, even scream, to get the fear out in the open, but I believe it is far healthier in the long run to release it that way, than to repress it with the 'help' of drugs and/or breathing exercises.

It is also important for you to feel that you can be powerful about dealing with your panicky feelings. After all, everything passes and feelings are just feelings. There is always a reason for feeling afraid; you just need to be able to get the release to handle it well. If you can let fear take its course, instead of fighting it, panicking at its first manifestation, you will be in charge, using its energy to change your life, instead of letting it overwhelm you.

Professional performers, such as actors, racing drivers, TV presenters, musicians, and barristers say they always have 'stage fright' and even shake and sweat throughout, but it doesn't stop them doing their jobs, and in many instances even enhances their performance, by giving them that extra surge of adrenalin that keeps them alert even when they know their part or the course so well that they could enact it in their sleep.

Jealousy/envy. When you feel jealousy or envy or both they are telling you what you really want. Jealousy is very much rooted in your frozen need for love, affection, validation from one special person (or more). The feeling that you cannot bear someone else to have the person you can't have, that you don't feel important enough, loved enough, IS YOUR FEELING. It usually has nothing to do with the other person (although there are people who use jealousy to manipulate others' emotions). Envy is usually a frozen need for things, achievements, consumer durables, gains, relationships which you feel you cannot have in your own right, for whatever reason.

Jealousy and envy draw on our core emotions of fear, anger and grief, and can be totally overwhelming. They can make you behave uncharacteristically, such as snooping on a loved ones' activities, reading their private letters and, in extreme cases, taking revenge. When you feel *jealous* you are really feeling powerless and deeply humiliated that 'you are not *the one*'. *Envy* is often based on greed – feeling you need to have everything all the time – which in turn is based on frozen needs to fill the yawning gap of insecurity.

The basic rules for releasing jealousy and envy are:

- Face and accept that you have these feelings, no matter how much your 'head' says you should not have them. We often deny these feelings intellectually because we feel ashamed to own up. Indeed, they can make you feel very vulnerable. You are showing someone that they matter to you, that you feel they have some power over you. In reality, they only have the power you give to them. You are no longer two years of age, even if you sometimes feel that you are.

- Release the feelings by talking in confidence to someone (a friend, counsellor, family member, trusted work colleague, priest, or Samaritan), about how you really feel. Release your unbridled desires verbally. Tell your listener what you want to do to the object of your desire, how small it makes you feel, how eaten up with revenge you are.

- Write jealous/envious letters – don't censor yourself at all. BUT DON'T SEND THEM. Keep them for a couple of weeks, then read them when you have cooled down. You will probably see a needy, lonely, misunderstood, affection-starved child looking back at you from the words. You may be relieved you didn't send the letters. If, however, you still feel revengeful, write some more, until you've got it out of your system. BUT DON'T SEND THEM. When you reach the stage where you can read through what you have written without feeling any strong emotion, simply tear them up. They have served their purpose. If you keep them – keep them private.

- On no account act on your feelings of revenge/pain, no matter how drawn you are to doing so (and these feelings can be overwhelmingly strong). Stories abound about jilted girlfriends making long-distance calls from the UK to Australia on their ex-lovers' phones or cutting up their partners' favourite suits. They are funny stories (we laugh to release our fear about doing the same or having it done to us), but they bring shame and indignity on to the shoulders of the avenger in question. Some people can feel driven to violence – DON'T SUCCUMB. Turn your anger, grief, humiliation to some good by bashing out your feelings on a punchball or squash court, where you can experience re-lease and keep fit at the same time. IT WON'T MAKE THEM LOVE YOU, NO MATTER WHAT YOU DO. (If you seek a destructive outlet, it will probably do just that – destroy.)

Boredom. This can be very irritating, debilitating, and frus-trating. It is a horrible emotion – feeling that you don't know what you want or what to do with yourself – and it is a major driving force behind addictions. Boredom is painful. It is also based on isolation and feeling unloved, as we saw in Chapter 2. How can you release boredom? Here are some suggestions:

- Recognize how you feel when you're bored: sexually frus-trated? Lethargic? Want to pick a fight? Destructive? Need to drive fast? Want to scream?

- Notice situations which make you feel bored. They are often where you are not engaged on any level (such as when in a meeting at work which doesn't impinge on your work area), or a family get-together (where you feel no-one is paying you enough attention), or during particular films, types of activity or, most commonly, having time on your hands. Get wise to what triggers your boredom.

- Decide to feel boredom rather than run from it. We try to distract ourselves when we feel bored, which often occasions a visit to the off-licence, taking drugs and/or making mischief of some sort (boredom is a key motivator behind smashed telephone boxes and similar vandalism – it is really a young person's way of saying 'Give me some attention. I'm bored, lonely, scared and don't know what to do with myself'). If you stop running from feeling boredom, you can start doing something about it instead.

- Tell someone – or write down how you feel. You may feel yourself becoming tearful or angry when you do; let it go, lose control, that's fine. Boredom is a mixture of emotions, so you will feel confused about how you feel precisely but you do know that you feel painfully bored. Getting attention from someone is the antidote.

- You do not need to rush to fill the space when you're bored. In fact, parents will know their children present all sorts of emotions when they are bored, which gives the parents a hard time trying to 'think of something to do'. Every suggestion may meet with a blank stare, or even a tantrum. It is far better to pay attention to the underlying feelings and allow the child to release them through raging, crying, stamping their foot, telling you how they really feel, rather than simply trying to distract them. Yet, this can be hard for parents to do because they are under pressure and probably can't imagine what it's like to have nothing to do and feel bored. However, above all, don't get angry with your child (or anyone else for that matter) for being bored. It is not their fault, and they are telling you that something is not right.

As a General Rule

By now, you will have seen a pattern emerging in the above, which can be applied to any other emotions you experience:

- Face the feelings.
- Accept the feelings.

- Release the feelings appropriately.

- Get help/support to continue facing, accepting and releasing feelings.

- Get wise to your own emotions.

- Give yourself what you need as if you are your own parent.

EMOTIONAL NOURISHMENT

Emotional nourishment is more than managing your feelings in everyday life, it is about feeding and nurturing yourself at a deep emotional level. Everyone needs emotional nourishment, even if you think you don't. There will come a time, perhaps a crisis such as a bereavement, redundancy, splitting up with a partner, when you will feel the need for emotional nourishment. But if you nurture your emotional needs as a matter of course, then crises and everyday problems won't seem so daunting. You will have built reliable resources to deal with things that come your way, and you will not be 'knocked sideways' in the same way that you would be otherwise.

How to Nourish Yourself Emotionally

Build your own boundaries. As we saw in Chapter 2: Facing and Releasing Your Emotions, and Chapter 5: Facing Relationships, this is *not* the same as saying put barriers up, keep everyone out and remain isolated. It means learn what is and what is not acceptable to you with other people, in terms of trust, intimacy, self-revelation and closeness. Keep some private space around you, so you can feel you are in charge of your emotional life.

Learn to be separate. Many of us have an 'urge to merge' with our family, partners, friends. This means we can't really distinguish the difference between 'us' and 'them', so we make assumptions about them, their motives, and their feelings. We invade their boundaries by telling them what to think, by bossing them about or manipulating them emotionally, or clinging on to them like needy babies in the most inappropriate ways. By learning to be separate you cease to 'double guess' everyone else's needs, and you cease to want to control other people's actions, feelings and thoughts. Instead, you can state what you want and you can listen to what they want. And if your individual wants turn out to be very different, that's fine. You can agree to differ, do things separately, or take time to think through the implications of any decision.

However, you do not have to persuade them to agree with you, threaten to leave them or punish them if they don't, or feel threatened by their wanting something entirely different. Compromises can be worked out with sensitivity and open talk, but you do not have to agree to something you don't want to. You may decide on a third, mutual course of action, which is completely different from the two you both thought of first.

If you separate your needs out from other people's it means you are entirely responsible for yourself and no-one else.

Be honest with yourself. But you don't have to be honest with everyone. This is a tricky one, as honesty and openness are held up as important, particularly by certain religions. However, there are times when it is pertinent or appropriate not to be honest. You don't have to tell Auntie Joan that you hate the Christmas present she gave you. You equally don't have to pretend you love it. But you can be politic – by saying 'thanks', smiling and leaving it at that.

In relationships, if you are a separate person, with boundaries, you can choose what you say to whom about what. You will have an inner life; you can have thoughts and feelings which are entirely your own. You can do things which are known only to you. However, you need to watch out if you are a secretive person who likes living in fantasy – because then you could be lying to yourself, rather than being honest. Ultimately, *you* know whether you are acting with integrity, whether you feel ashamed or guilty, because you know when what you are doing 'goes against the grain'. This means understanding the kind of person you are and how to operate in the world with aware honesty.

End self-sabotage. Sometimes we think or behave in ways that are the complete opposite of what we really want deep inside. You may want to get close to someone, but you push them away instead. You may want to get a new job, but fail to fill in the application forms and get them in on time. This is self-sabotage. We can commit it in all sorts of ways and, really, it is just old fear taking over. Keep your eyes open for where you trip yourself up on your own obstacle course. Remove the obstacles by ending self-sabotage and life will be much more emotionally fulfilling.

Love yourself actively – and continue building your self-esteem. Here are some of the ways in which you can do this:

- Keep noticing what is right about you instead of what's wrong with you.

- Continue adding to your notebook lists of what you like/ love about yourself, what you do well, who loves you.

- Allow yourself pleasure in life everyday without harming yourself, making addictive 'treats' redundant. (For more on this, see the following Chapters, especially Chapters 11-18).

- Reach out and get support, help and advice when you need it.

- Learn to listen well without making judgements and comparisons.

- Learn to take your turn at talking, with appropriate levels of intimacy.

- Give up gossip, moaning, being mean, taking revenge, all of which are powerless pursuits which eat into your integrity and personal strength.

- Choose what you do to your body. Be aware of chemical and emotional addictions and when you're on the Addictive Treadmill. Decide to step off and look at how you are really feeling instead.

- Don't go to the shoe shop for bread. In other words, go to the shoe shop for shoes and bread shop for bread. We often try to get emotional nourishment from the very people, activities and habits who/which provide the opposite. Notice who cares for you, thinks well about you, listens to you. Notice what nourishes you rather than depletes your energy and go to these sources instead. Trust those who are trustworthy – don't trust those who are unreliable, liars, ungenerous and deeply hurt themselves.

- Give up the notion that you are 'a hopeless case', a 'failure' or that 'nobody likes you'. If you think that, it may be true because of what you project into the world.

- 'Act as if' you are irresistible, fun to be with, intelligent, lovable, worthy of good things, deserving, a success, and you will be.

- Remember that you are imperfect – and that that is fine. You are human, you can make mistakes (and rectify them like a grown up). Perfection is neither achievable nor desirable. Being a bit flawed is much more attractive, lovable and real.

- Accept yourself for who and what you are – unique, original, human – just you.

- Live in the present and give up regret. You will get more satisfaction from everyday life if you do.

Getting back in touch with reality. Sometimes you can feel 'sunk' in depression. You need to learn to get yourself back in touch with reality at these times, even though it can feel virtually impossible. Some useful tips:

- Make a scrap book and fill it with your favourite pictures, photos and memorabilia, and if you feel low flick through it, reminding yourself of good times and people in your life.

- Go round your home, garden and neighbourhood and notice things that are good to look at: flowers, trees, colours, smells, animals, shapes of buildings, the sky, pictures, furniture you like.

- Remind yourself of some 'good early memories' connected with easy pleasures such as swimming, walking, playing, eating, the seaside, holidays. It is good to do this with a buddy, or partner. Ask each other, 'what is a good early memory of . . .' and fill in the dots. Take it in turns to ask the questions and to answer.

These exercises are designed to bring your attention back to reality and away from being stuck in your distress.

DIRECTION FOR MEETING YOUR EMOTIONAL NEEDS

Finally, two directions that work very well are to say the following as often as you can (at least 10 times daily):

'From this moment on I decide to give up abusing myself in any way at all, and instead, I will love and forgive myself completely, I will cherish my mind and my body, I will remember that I'm good and intelligent and all I need do is to simply relax and enjoy myself because I'm alive. This means. . .' Fill in your notebook with your first thoughts.

....

....

'I will not give in to the ancient and addictive pull to feel and communicate how lonely and miserable I am in the hope of getting help. It never worked anyway. So I now decide to remember — and act on the knowledge — that I am already completely happy, have a very good life, can be my own parent and have absolutely everything going for me. This means . . .' Fill in your notebook with your first thoughts.

....

....

Chapter 11

———■○■———

Meeting Your Physical Needs

So far we have been looking at how you can be your own parent by meeting your emotional needs to overcome your addictions. Equally important is meeting your physical needs. Of course, there is an overlap between the two. For instance, you may crave a cup of tea because, emotionally, it allows you a ten minute rest and/or social time in a busy day, and makes you feel cared for. At the same time, if you are a regular tea-drinker, you will probably have a physical dependence on caffeine (the main stimulant in tea), which you only notice when you don't drink as much as usual and perhaps suffer withdrawal symptoms, such as headaches, tiredness and nausea.

THE MIND-BODY LINK

Over the past 20 years there has been increasing public interest in the extent to which our psychological well-being affects our physical health: in other words, the mind-body link. Mainstream medical professionals are more aware today of the impact of depression, bereavement and other traumas on health, and take these factors into account when diagnosing and prescribing. No longer writing repeat prescriptions for tranquillizers and sleeping pills so readily, doctors have become aware of how negative emotions can weaken health. And one positive result of the AIDS crisis has been to make us all more immune-system and health conscious.

As a culture we are no longer looking at illness as a purely physical phenomenon and the belief that a healthy mind leads to a healthy body has never been so prevalent. At the same time, vegetarianism and alternative health therapies such as homeopathy, acupuncture, shiatsu, aromatherapy, osteopathy, hypnosis, once thought to be the sole preserve of 'health freaks', are now virtually mainstream. Nearly every chemist can provide alternative as well as allopathic (traditional) medicines, and some GPs and Consultants refer patients to alternative remedies, practitioners and even homoeopathic hospitals. A few GPs practise both types of health care.

The 'fitness boom' of the 1980s and 1990s has brought about greater public awareness of the necessity for good nutrition. While there has been a lot of confusion over cholesterol, eggs, additives to poultry, meat and canned foods and BSE, there has also been a general trend towards healthier eating. The rise in consumption of non- and low-alcoholic drinks, low-tar cigarettes, decaffeinated tea and coffee, herb teas and sugar-free soft drinks, reflect public concern about everyday drug-intake.

Also, women are having babies later – and need to keep themselves fit longer for motherhood. The detrimental impact upon foetuses of chemicals from smoking, antibiotics and alcohol is now common knowledge. We generally want to look better, feel healthier, live longer, be fitter and have more choices and fun.

Meanwhile, addiction continues to be both a private and public blot on the nation's health. We may feel that it is on the increase – which in some areas, such as alcohol consumption – it is. Yet, we are more aware of the dangers of physical and psychological harm than ever before. And eating disorders, such as anorexia and bulimia nervosa, have become everyday terms due to the revelations about the late Princess Diana's private hell. If Royalty has been able to unstiffen its upper lip and seek professional help, then surely there's hope for the rest of us to be able to do something about similar problems!

YOUR PHYSICAL NEEDS

So what are your physical needs? What do you struggle with, feel hopeless about, feel powerless to change physically? Remembering that the way to get off the hook is to meet your real needs, rather than try to fill your frozen needs, jot down in your notebook what you think your physical needs are.

....

....

Do you meet your physical needs for yourself currently? Or are you waiting for the right time to start? Perhaps you feel that you don't know enough to begin? Whatever, you will not be able to give up your addiction until you pay some attention to this area of your life. Doing so may well bring up feelings, in which case, refer back to Chapter 10: Meeting Your Emotional Needs, and release those feelings. That way, you stay in charge and increase your personal empowerment.

This chapter will not give you all the answers, but it may help you to pinpoint your own physical needs in more details so you can begin to get to grips with meeting them.

EATING DISORDERS

We all have to eat to live, and eating disorders are possibly the hardest types of addiction to tackle because your relationship with food goes back right to the beginning of your life. You may have an addiction to not eating and literally starving yourself through compulsive dieting, and/or anorexia nervosa. Or you might be compulsively eating, stuffing yourself during 'binges' with whatever food meets your particular needs. If you make yourself sick after a binge, you may have bulimia nervosa.

It is currently estimated that 90 per cent of people with eating disorders are women, 10 per cent are men. But, overall, the proportion of people with eating disorders is going up – and so is the number of male sufferers. Also both anorexia and bulimia have been identified among children, particularly girls. The onset of menstruation is one of the most vulnerable times, especially for anorexia, because of the fear a developing sexuality can create in girls and young women. Anorexia becomes a self-abusive way of exercising control over your own body and of keeping it childlike and underdeveloped (for instance, periods often stop), through starvation.

Why is Eating Such a Problem?

- We learn habits from our parents, so if you have a parent with an eating disorder, you will have seen strange eating patterns and attitudes as 'normal' and probably copied them.

- Your culture will have given you beliefs about food. A poor family might experience food as being scarce, so there might be competition and fighting over it, an urge to eat whenever you can, and never waste a scrap – even if your hunger has already been satisfied.

- Men are often thought of as more 'deserving' of food because they supposedly go out and do rugged work to support a family. So, men can get the best and women and children take second best. This can be carried on into adult life.

- We are given 'treats' in childhood to shape our behaviour and make us 'good', so we learn to reward ourselves with sugary things, like chocolate, sweets, cakes, ice-cream, biscuits, puddings and this special 'treat' value continues into adulthood.

- We have all eaten a lot of sugar inadvertently, through baby foods, tinned and processed foods, soft drinks and snacks – so you can get addicted to sugar without realizing it.

- If you feel bad about yourself in any way – depressed, or sad, or angry – you may use food (or the absence of it) as a way of dealing with difficult and painful emotions. You learn to use food as 'punishment' or 'reward'. You may comfort yourself with food, or deny yourself. There is a very strong emotional aspect to eating disorders, so they can also be a response to childhood neglect or abuse. If you feel scared and lonely, eating too much or too little can be a way of trying to numb painful feelings. We can also refuse food and be very fussy about it as a form of rebellion, or to attract attention.

What You Can Do About Eating Disorders

Own up to having an eating problem – and you are already on your way to getting off the hook.

Decide to take control of your eating. Be your own parent, and learn to nourish yourself. Believe that you are worth feeding properly and well. This can be very difficult, but you *can* do it.

Inform yourself. Read about your difficulty with food. Women's magazines, bookshops, libraries, health stores and alternative health therapy centres are invaluable sources of information (see also 'Help' section for sources).

Remember that you are not alone. Millions of people suffer from eating disorders. You might join a support group through the Eating Disorders Association (EDA) (see 'Help' section), and read the EDA magazine, *Signpost*. It can be very helpful to talk to others who are going through or have been through similar problems.

Get counselling help.   Sometimes it is useful to talk to someone objective, but empathetic, when beginning to deal with your feelings. You can find counsellors in your area through the EDA.

Get your attention off food.   Stop worrying about what you eat. I *know* this is easier said than done, but being completely focused on food problems often masks deeper emotional difficulties, such as fear of intimacy or getting on with your life. Try to make progress in other spheres, such as changing your job, cleaning out chaotic cupboards or generally improving your home environment. It will boost your self-esteem to be able to do something to help yourself, even if it's not directly to do with food.

Decide to change your eating habits.   Eat regularly and well, in order to nourish yourself. You have probably never learned to do this, for various reasons, but you deserve it. Learn to eat a balanced diet and make a timetable for each day, outlining what you will eat and when, with other activities in between.

Make contact with other people.   This is especially important when you start to change your eating habits. If you have a counsellor, talk to him or her first. You could also ask your GP to refer you to an NHS dietician. Then decide which of your friends, family, or work colleagues might be supportive. It can be very frightening to own up to what you really do, but it can also be wonderful to have someone on your side who really understands.

• If you're a starver you will need to learn to take in nourishment, that you deserve it, that it's good to be alive. Start with very small amounts of tempting and delicious foods. Simply eat regularly. Set an alarm clock or timer to remind you if you don't have reliable hunger pangs. Start noticing feelings of hunger as they arise and respond to them by having something to eat. You may still not feel hungry at 'meal times' – that's fine. Just remember, you are worth feeding and try to eat at least a small amount.

- If you are a stuffer you will need to be aware of the feeling that something has to take the place of your favourite addiction. You may feel a huge, yawning gap and a lot of fear about not filling it, but it is just fear and if you can release it, you can begin to adjust fairly quickly without recourse to substitute addictions. You'll definitely feel better about not stuffing yourself, which will boost your self-esteem.

Accept your body.   A lot of eating disorders are to do with not accepting either your body or your sexuality. You probably don't feel too good about your appearance and you may feel 'if only' something was better about your physique the whole of your life would be changed. This is an illusion. Only internal change can make a difference long term. Losing that stone in weight WON'T bring the perfect person into your life. All the plastic surgery in the world can't stop you ageing or being who you are. So accept yourself.

DIET AND NUTRITION

It is important to treat yourself well by paying attention to your diet – you are what you eat. Popping the odd vitamin pill won't do much for you if you are living on TV dinners, pot noodles, chocolate and crisps. But it can be very confusing to work out which diet is best for you as there are so many to choose from.

You might also feel that you haven't got the time to invest in changing your diet. Or, even if you want to eat organic vegetables and fruit, you might fear the expense. Or you may well be worried by the fact that agriculture is leaning heavily on chemicals and even our drinking water has become unappetizing, so we have turned to mineral water instead.

On the plus side, British cuisine has become a lot more cosmopolitan: in addition to our own standard fare, we eat Italian, Greek, Chinese, French, Indian, Mexican and US foods, thus increasing the variety and interest in food. At the same time, the old 'chips and . . .' diet persists in many households. What we have gained in variety and nutritional knowledge, we have often lost in purity and goodness. Yet, we now know there is a need for a general low-salt, low-sugar or sugar-free, low-fat, additive-free diet.

How to Improve Your Diet

You will need your notebook again, this time to study what you eat and drink. When it is all down in black and white you will have a clear picture of how healthy your present diet is – and where you need to make improvements.

1. Keep a food 'diary' for a week: write down everything you eat and drink during the day and when you eat or drink it. Notice the times when you run out of energy and pop into the kitchen to make a piece of toast and cup of tea, or slip out from work to buy a chocolate bar to 'keep you going'. You have your own energy levels and biorhythms – and it's important to notice what they are so you can be prepared to meet them.

2. Note HOW you eat, why or when. Do you sit down and eat at a table in a relaxed way? Or do you eat in front of the TV? Are you always on the run with a Mars Bar in your hand? Do you end up rowing with the family at mealtimes? Or do you always sit down in peace, chew slowly and really taste your food?

3. Notice how much sugar, chocolate, fat, fast foods, soft drinks, snacks (crisps, peanuts, etcetera), you consume.

4. Do you graze? That is, do you snack all day without having a proper meal? Grazing is increasingly popular with busy people eating on the run – but it's not good for your digestion, and can lead to stomach ulcers and poor nutrition.

5. How much fresh fruit and vegetables do you eat? Could you eat more? Do you rely on tinned fruit and vegetables? And if so, could you use a healthier alternative?

   ....

6. How much caffeine do you drink in the form of tea, coffee, cola and other soft drinks?

   ....

7. If you have periods, do you crave chocolate when pre-menstrual? Do you find yourself eating more at that time of the month?

   ....

8. Do you ever miss meals and drink alcohol instead? And/or do you go out drinking and eat large meals (especially take-aways) late at night, to soak up alcohol?

   ....

9. Do you eat when you're actually hungry or when you think you *should* eat (because it's a meal-time)?

   ....

10. Do you tend to live on processed foods because you 'can't be bothered' to cook after a busy day at work and/or caring for children?

    ....

A Balanced Diet

It is very important to learn what you need to eat in order to sustain good health, high energy levels and balance in your diet. I'm not going to prescribe what you eat – rather I'm going to suggest some general guidelines for improvement. You will need to take into account your own personal needs related to your: budget, culture, religion (i.e. rules for food preparation), lifestyle (i.e. whether you work shifts, work part-time, eat with the children, eat out on business, etc), allergies, availability of foodstuffs, individual taste, individual metabolism (i.e. how fast you 'burn up' food).

If you follow these basic guidelines you will improve your diet and nourish yourself properly, making the use of chemical and emotional addictions which give you 'trash energy' less attractive:

Be realistic. Don't adopt an elaborate and unworkable diet that takes hours to prepare (unless you want to, for pleasure). Work out how much time you've got available and plan your meals accordingly.

Be organized. You don't have to be a supercook, but if you know you get hungry at work during the morning and afternoon, then take healthy snacks with you: fresh or dried fruit, unsalted nuts, carrot sticks, etcetera. If you know you feel like eating late at night, get in some healthy foods, like yoghurt, fruit, wholemeal bread. Make sure you have in store adequate supplies of healthy food for a week. That way you will be less tempted to stave off hunger with chocolate, biscuits and fast foods. If you have a freezer, stock up on healthy foods such as batch-cooked soups, stews, fish, which you can use at short notice.

Be prepared. If you need to get something out of the freezer to cook, get it out in the morning, or a few hours before. Have some basics to hand, like cheese, salad, pitta bread, fish cakes, veggie burgers, so if someone pops in to see you, you can quickly prepare a healthy snack. If you plan to cook with pulses and beans, allow enough time to soak and boil them, so you do not have to resort to using additive/sugar/salt-stacked canned or processed foods.

Buy organic and free range. If possible, include some organic vegetables, fruit and dairy produce in your diet, to reduce the amounts of toxins you take in from pesticides, etcetera. You can get free-range chicken, bacon, eggs, milk, cheese, yoghurt (and organic vegetables and fruit) from most large supermarket chains now. If you eat beef check it's organic and from young stock.

Be careful. With cook-chill foods, using a microwave, storing food, read the instructions carefully. It is easy to be careless about cooking times, not defrosting frozen foods properly, and storing foods haphazardly. Store cooked and raw foods separately and always cover dishes of left-overs in the fridge. Never store foods in open cans as they go off quickly. Watch sell-by dates and stick to them. Carefully date-label foods you have prepared at home for freezing. Keep your cooking areas, fridge, microwave and freezer clean. And keep pet foods and dishes separate from your food. Don't put yourself at risk unnecessarily from salmonella or E. Coli poisoning.

Specific Tips About Diet

To overcome your addictions completely, you need to be well-nourished. Here are some useful dietary tips:

Low or no salt. There is plenty of salt in everyday foods. If you *must* add salt, use sea- or bio-salt. But leave it out if you can, your palate will adjust quickly and your heart will benefit.

Cut out refined sugar – or use non-saccharine substitutes. If you have a sweet tooth, then try fructose, the naturally occurring sugar found in fresh fruit, honey or maple syrup (but remember they are still sugars). You can now get sugar-free ice-creams and soft-drinks.

High-fibre reduces the risk of cancer – of the bowel and colon. So use whole, brown rice and pasta, flour, grains and cereals. Add a little bran to porridge and muesli for extra fibre.

Eat fresh fruit and vegetables daily – preferably raw or only lightly cooked. Wash fruit and vegetables thoroughly to reduce pesticide intake. Cook vegetables gently, such as by steaming them so they remain crunchy and full of vitamins. Or cook them in their own liquids, covered with tin foil in a dish in the oven or microwave, dotted with a few knobs of low-fat margarine and/or a little olive oil.

Eat at least five servings of fruit or vegetables a day. Eat some salad – including leafy, dark green salad vegetables such as watercress and spinach – at least once a day. There are many different types of lettuce on the market today, so salads needn't be boring. Make simple dressings from extra-virgin olive oil (no cholesterol), lemon juice, fresh basil leaves, crushed garlic and black pepper. Add a dash of Dijon mustard for bite.

'Snack' on high-fibre fillers – such as fruit and nuts, trail mixes, crunchy cereal and dried fruit bars (look for sugar-free ones), dried fruits, or fresh fruit, carrot sticks.

Low or no fat. You can get low or no fat cheeses, yoghurt, fromage frais, Quark, margarines. You can also use soya bean based products, such as tofu and soya milk, which are excellent sources of protein. Avoid genetically modified foods.

Meat. If you are a meat-eater, limit your intake of lean red meat to once a week (try organic, free-range meat to reduce your intake of antibiotics and other drugs). If possible, eat only lean bacon, and free-range, corn-fed chickens.

Fish. Eat fish twice a week (if you like fish). Go for oily fish such as mackerel, herrings, trout, salmon, tuna and white fish, such as cod, plaice. Ask where your seafood has come from and avoid North Sea fish because of pollution.

Eggs. Use free range, if you eat eggs. Because of their cholesterol content it is also best to limit your intake to three or four a week. Opt for two- not three-egg omelettes. Don't forget that rich sauces, such as Hollandaise and Bearnaise, and mayonnaise, usually contain a lot of cholesterol because of the ingredients: eggs, cream, butter, milk, oil, etcetera.

Alcohol. Watch your intake, if you drink. Recommended weekly limits are 14 units for women, 21 units for men. One unit is half a pint of beer, OR one glass of wine, OR one shot of spirits. Keep track of your drinking and alternate with mineral water and soft drinks. Don't drink every day; give your liver and kidneys a rest. If you do drink alcohol, drink lots of water before bedtime to counteract dehydration. Remember, alcohol is 'empty calories', so don't give up eating in favour of drinking. You can also try de-alcoholized or low alcohol wines, ciders and beers, which give you the taste of alcohol, without the buzz.

Drink 2 to 3 litres of water a day (preferably filtered or mineral). This helps to detoxify your system.

Overall, it is important to *enjoy* eating and drinking. Always eat when you are sitting down – preferably at the table. Make your eating environment relaxing with candles, flowers and music. Present your food attractively, take time to relish its flavours, eat slowly. Rushing along the high-street gobbling high-cholesterol junk food isn't treating yourself with the respect you deserve.

ENERGY AND THE IMMUNE SYSTEM

Energy is essential for a strong immune system, and comes from properly nourishing ourselves. Energy is our life force, it keeps us from getting ill, enables us to work and play, and is often the main characteristic that other people notice about us. When we talk about someone being 'radiant', 'enthusiastic', 'fun to be with', 'positive' or 'exciting', we are actually describing their energy levels. In fact, the existence of energy can be measured by 'Kirlian photography', a scientific process which records people's energy fields on special magnetized plates. Kirlian pictures show energy as patterns and colours emanating from limbs, such as hands or feet.

When we feel we're becoming ill, we often feel 'below par', 'off colour' or 'drained', and we may have a rest or go on holiday to 'recharge our batteries'. These terms reveal that feeling of low energy which occurs just before and during illness, when your immune system is weakened. In other words, when your energy levels are depleted, for whatever reason, your immune system ceases to protect you and you get sick.

Maximizing our energy levels has become a major focus, especially in the food and pharmaceutical industries, where products are marketed on (sometimes bogus) claims of increasing energy. This can mean that they contain sugar or glucose, or a synthetic drug, such as caffeine, meant to 'boost' your energy levels. In actual fact, such products deplete your body's resources because they're 'trash energy', which means you may feel pepped, or speeded, up for a while, but then you crash, and need to have another dose to keep going.

In other words, you are back on the Addictive Treadmill again, and as a result you can feel very exhausted, irritable and flat. So it is better to try to boost your energy levels without cups of caffeine-laden coffee and bars of sweet chocolate, and keep yourself going by healthier means, such as mineral water or herb teas, and fresh fruit or vegetable crudités.

How to Boost Your Energy and Improve Your Immune System

Relaxation. It is important to build periods of rest and relaxation into every day. You can also meditate, which helps slow your mind and body down, allowing you to relax deeply. Even five minutes with your mind 'switched off' and your feet up can boost your energy significantly. Ideally, you should aim for an hour a day, say, half an hour morning and evening. If you really can't do that – try for 15 minutes at each end of the day. You could also use train and bus journeys as relaxation time. (For simple relaxation techniques, turn to Relaxation and Sleep, later in this chapter.)

Healthy diet. A primary source of energy is a healthy diet. Energy/immune-system-boosting foods are: carbohydrates such as bread, cereals, pasta, nuts and seeds, rice and grains); fresh vegetables (such as broccoli, spinach, watercress, potatoes, garlic, onions, sprouts, carrots); protein (fish, lean red meat); dairy produce (cheese, eggs); soya products (such as tofu); and fresh fruit (such as oranges, apples, pears, grapefruit, bananas). It is especially important not to eat on the run, Big Mac in hand, and *never* 'crash diet' to lose weight for a special occasion. (See Diet and Nutrition, page 174.)

Regular exercise.   When we get home from work exhausted or feel frazzled after a day with the children, exercise can seem the least attractive option and instead, we slump in front of the TV. Yet, when you're feeling drained, half an hour of vigorous exercise can boost your energy much more than a cuppa and biscuit consumed while comfortably watching your favourite soap opera. When at work, going for a quick walk round the block or upstairs to another office, will oxygenate your bloodstream and perk you up. If you've got limited time, half an hour non-stop swimming is good. Even housework, such as hoovering or cleaning, even cutting the grass or hedge, is good, healthy exercise.

If you take up sport, make sure you think about your body's needs and any possible vulnerable points. Take professional advice from your GP, or a personal fitness trainer and/or your local sports centre, gym or health club, etc. (See Exercise and Fitness opposite.)

Sleep.   Getting enough sleep can be difficult if you work and play hard, or are bringing up young children. But adequate sleep is essential if you want to keep your energy/immune system levels high. Everyone's needs are different, but make sure you get enough (making sure, however, that you don't use sleep as an escape from facing difficulties). Some people find 'cat naps' give them extra energy, and can drop off for 'forty winks' whenever they want. Others need longer naps in the afternoon, after lunch, when energy levels dip. (See Sleep, page 194.)

Alternative health therapies.   Alternative health therapies, and/or holistic medicine, aim to boost the body's vital energy by creating internal balance. Therapies, such as acupuncture, shiatsu, homeopathy, reflexology can have a very positive, long-lasting impact on the body's immune system. (See 'Help' section for useful contacts and reading.)

EXERCISE AND FITNESS

As we have already seen, exercise is important to boost your energy and immune system. But if you've been a sloth until now fitness can only be attained gradually – so do not rush headlong into a tortuous regime. Choose an exercise plan that fits into your life, rather than dominates it (you may well be escaping something that is emotionally difficult to face, if you become an exercise fanatic).

Some General Guidelines

These might be helpful for you when working out what exercise to take up. Make sure you take all your physical needs into account:

Exercise every week.   Walk to the post office or down to the shops instead of taking the car. Walk up and down stairs instead of using the lift. Write in your diary when you are going swimming or meeting a friend for a game of squash or walking the dog in the park. That way you will make exercise as important as all your other commitments, and you can see at a glance whether you are taking enough, regular exercise.

Get professional advice – about what sports/exercise will suit your physical abilities. Talk to your doctor, your local leisure centre, health club, gym and/or phone up your local council for advice (under Leisure Services). Some clubs now have 'personal fitness trainers' who can advise you on a tailor-made exercise regime. Even better (but more expensive) you can hire a personal fitness trainer (contact the YMCA in London; address in 'Help' section). If you find it hard to get yourself to do any exercise on your own, make a date with a friend and work out together. You could also do structured exercises at home, using a video; if you are shy about showing yourself in public this is a good way to start.

Be realistic.   Work out an exercise plan that suits your life, your pocket, your hours, your family and social life, your age and fitness levels and, of course, your body's needs (your heart, back, lungs, etc). Don't make exercise a strain and a pain. Don't go for 'the burn', as you can do yourself serious damage. Warm up at the beginning of any exercise session and wind down at the end (this should be built in by the trainer – so be careful to stick to the prescribed routine if you repeat the exercises at home). Try gentle but very efficient all over body exercise, such as swimming. Try new sports, too; don't say you can't do them before you've even tried.

Be gentle on yourself.   Use exercise as a way of pleasuring yourself. Take along gorgeous-smelling hair and body shampoos and body lotions. Pamper yourself: you should feel nurtured, pleasantly tingly, and relaxed afterwards. Exercise is supposed to be a treat, a way of stretching and toning yourself, not a spartan punishment to be endured.

Be sociable.   Exercise and sport is a great way of meeting people. If you are single and want to meet new people, take up a team sport, like volleyball, rather than swimming or jogging alone. Don't change and rush off afterwards; have a drink or something to eat with other players. If you want to make friends, don't wait for someone else to suggest it – take the initiative.

Don't become addicted.   Exercise can be a very good way of working out anger, frustration and pain. Some people find running round a field or a tennis court or smashing a ball with a bat an immensely satisfying way of dealing with feelings. But beware of exercise becoming an addiction in itself. This can happen if you become obsessed with your sport, having to do it longer each day, more frequently, to the point where you have no social, private or family life left. Anything you do compulsively, and to the exclusion of balance in your life, can lead you on to the Addictive Treadmill.

If you are hurt emotionally, you will need to face what is going on underneath at some point. Disappearing to the gym every time life gets tough is OK – up to a point – but if you never get to sort things out with people, face to face, then you could be missing out on the richness of human relationships and be staying stuck in your own isolation. If you think you might be addicted to exercise, turn back to Chapter 2 and Chapter 10, and think about how you can start meeting your real emotional needs.

Don't neglect your family, children, friends and partners through your sport. It's fine to withdraw into your exercise world occasionally, but if you do it all the time – then something's wrong probably. Be thoughtful about the amount you exercise, and whom it affects in your life – make sure you spend time with the people that you might be running away from rather than face up to relationship problems and resolve them. Stop and think how it feels to be in a relationship with you. Would *you* like it?

Of course, if you are a professional athlete and competing at the highest levels, or wanting to be one, you will have to put in hours of dedicated training. But most of us are amateurs, striving for our 'personal best'. If you are living, breathing, eating your sport, you may be avoiding intimacy, closeness and responsibility at home.

Most of all – enjoy yourself! Exercise can be fun. It's supposed to be a life-enhancing, pleasurable activity, not a matter of life or death. Your self-esteem doesn't hang entirely on whether or not you win at badminton. A sporting attitude is one of being thoroughly engaged during the activity and delighted with the outcome, whether or not you are the victor. Don't get sulky about losing. It is bad grace and you lose friends and self-respect. Be generous about other people's good skill and good fortune; that will nourish *you* as well. At the same time, you can set yourself personal challenges and meet them – which will boost your self-esteem. But try not to get rigid: if you want to swim 50 lengths, but 30 feels about right, stop there. Being your own parent on the exercise and fitness front means, do it; but don't over do it. Balance is all.

RELAXATION AND SLEEP

It is so easy to say: 'Relax!' and yet it can be so hard to do. Furthermore, what you usually think of as relaxation often includes addiction in some way. You might go out and get 'high' on alcohol and drugs to wind down. You might go out and find somebody to seduce. You might eat a 'slap up' meal, washed down by too much alcohol. You might watch TV until your eyes drop out. You might go on a spending spree, or drive the car along a motorway at high speed, in order to release tension. Of course, there is nothing wrong with any of these activities (unless you put yourself and others in serious danger) but there is something wrong when the ONLY means of relaxation you use involves chemical or emotional addiction.

Give Up Self-Abuse

If you take a decision to give up all forms of self-abuse (see Chapter 10 for advice), then you will have to find other ways to unwind.

Whatever you do:

- You will need to do it slowly and in moderation.

- You will need to be patient, because it takes time for any form of relaxation to start working.

- You will need to be flexible, because sometimes your schedule may get thrown by unforeseen circumstances.

- You will need to try things out and keep aware of how you really feel. Not everything will suit you, so experiment.

- You will need to make time to relax. You might feel you haven't got time, and keep putting it off. The irony is that if you make time to relax, the time you have got left tends to expand, and because you feel in better shape with more energy, daily tasks feel more manageable. So don't short-change yourself.

- You will feel more feelings, especially if you have usually used addictions to relax. Just accept you are going to feel them, whatever they are; they are just feelings and they will not damage you. Everything passes, including moods, upsets, excitement.

How to Relax

Develop a personal programme of relaxation which fits comfortably into your life. There is no perfect formula for relaxation, but the first step is to accept that you need to relax, without using addictions which can hurt you. Think about your lifestyle, budget, timetable, locality, physical ability, and personal preference. Relaxation techniques should be manageable, not a burden.

The following suggestions may help you to relax:

Waking up.   Don't just jump straight out of bed. Spend a few minutes stretching and yawning. Lie on your back, straight in bed, stretch your arms out above your head, point your toes – and stretch. Feel your spine stretching, feel your lungs filling with air, relax your jaw and let yourself yawn. Then roll on your side, bring your knees up towards your chest, and walk your hands along the bed towards you. Then sit upright. Gently swing your legs over the side of the bed and sit for a minute 'coming to', before getting up and on with the day.

Bathing and showering.   This can be wonderful, morning, noon or night. Don't stint yourself. Baths are more relaxing, because you can soak. You can buy wonderful perfumed oils and moisturizing lotions. Look out for aromatherapy oils which relax you, such as Basil, Lavender, Ylang-Ylang, Marjoram or Melissa. If you can, put half an hour aside, light a couple of safely-positioned candles, then switch off the electric light, put on soothing music using a portable radio or cassette player, sink your shoulders under the water level, with your head cushioned by a bath pillow (available from large chemists and department stores), and breathe in the warm, steamy aroma. Before you get out massage your body all over with soap, loofering away any hard skin and getting your circulation going.

If you have a partner, why not have a luxurious bath together? You can soap and massage each other, then sink back and soak in the warmth. Be sensual with each other, laugh and play. Why not get some toys for the bath, such as ducks and boats? You may begin to feel sexual, and that is fine, but try to stay with relaxing and playing on a 'fun' level.

Emotional release. If you are feeling tense at work, go into the loo and stretch and yawn, let yourself shiver if you feel a bit scared or 'upset'. Having a cry, even for five minutes, can relieve a lot of tension. If you're at home alone and feeling sad, put on a favourite cassette, get the Kleenex, cuddle a teddy bear, cushion or the cat, and let yourself go. If there's someone around, you could ask them to cuddle you for five minutes and let you cry. Explain that there's nothing wrong, you just need to be held. This can work wonders. You can also get into bed or into the bath to cry. When you feel a tautness in your chest and tears welling up, then it is time to cry. It's a great stress-reliever.

You might need to vent your anger. You need safety and privacy for this, so think about the neighbours and who else is around. It is best to let them know you are going to make some loud noises, otherwise it can really scare people. Get a big floor cushion, or two pillows or several small cushions, and pile them on the floor. Kneel, make a fist and with all your strength bash the cushions (you may feel detached and self-conscious at first), but keep bashing away and say or shout 'no' as vehemently as you can. If there is a problem with noise, you can stand up, shout 'no' or 'go away' into a cushion and stamp your feet in rage.

If you need to rip things, use old telephone directories. Avoid breaking objects and smashing up the place; this just leads to more grief and complications. And never direct your anger at someone else. It is your anger, not theirs. But you will feel a lot more relaxed, even exhausted, once you have let go some of your strong, bottled-up feelings.

Relaxation Techniques

There are many different relaxation techniques. You could take up Yoga or meditation. There may be a course at your local authority leisure centre or your local gym/health club. You might buy a video tape to help you relax. You can also get sounds of the rain-forest or sea sounds on cassette, which are immensely relaxing.

Here is a simple relaxation technique (which borrows from the Alexander Technique):

Allow yourself about half an hour for this exercise (set a timer or alarm clock). Choose a room distanced from the phone and any outside disturbances. Make sure also that you're not in a draught. Lock the door (if you can) and take off your shoes. Loosen any tight clothing (it's good to do this exercise in a track suit or leggings and T-shirt). Turn down the lighting, or draw the curtains, so the room is dimly lit.

- Place two paperback books one on top of the other on the floor to form a 'pillow'. Lie down, with the books under your head (your neck should be free) and pay attention to your lower back, which should be meeting the floor. To do this, bend your knees with your feet still on the ground, and as wide apart as the width of your pelvis. Put your arms by your sides, palms down, then bend them at the elbow and bring both your hands palms down on your chest (this should open your chest out).

- Close your eyes and take a few deep breaths. For a moment, notice the sounds of the outside world, and then ignore them. Think of your body as a big blancmange, sinking down into the floor, spreading in a jelly-like form.

- Notice your jaw and its tensions – let it sag. Be aware of your breathing, let it get deeper, breathing from your stomach, not just your chest.

- Now direct all your attention to your left foot, starting with the toes. Don't wiggle them, just 'feel' them from inside, one toe after the other.

- Now feel the rest of your foot: your heel pressing into the floor, the sole, the instep. Now imagine the whole foot being very heavy and sinking into the floor.

- Move on to the ankle – feel its shape; then up to the calf – tense it, and then relax it.

- Then move on to your kneecap, thigh, hip – tighten them up and then let them sink back into the floor. Notice the difference between how your left and right leg feel, before repeating the same technique with your right leg.

Having 'relaxed' both legs, go on to relax your whole body in the same way, following the order given below:

- pelvis

- lower back

- spine

- chest

- shoulders

- left arm (upper, elbow, forearm, wrist)

- left hand (palm, thumb, fingers)

- right arm and hand as above

- stomach

- face (eyes, jaws, mouth, tongue)

Finally, just let the whole of your body 'sink' through the floor. You should be very relaxed by now. Let any thoughts or feelings simply float through your mind and out again – just LET GO.

When your timer goes off – don't stir yourself abruptly. Roll over on to one side, bring your knees up towards your chest, and walk your hands along the floor, palms down, with your body facing forwards until you're upright. Sit for a minute, then get up slowly, avoiding putting strain on your lower back. Don't jump back into your everyday routine straightaway.

RELAXATION AT WORK

Because most of us spend eight hours a day at work, it is important to be able to 'turn off' for a while.

It increases productivity overall and lessens wear and tear on you. You can use your lunchtimes and tea breaks to relax. Skip the tea, coffee, crisps, fizzy drinks and sweet foods and go to the staff rest room (if you have one) or the cloakroom, or outside to get some fresh air. You can also do some exercises at your desk to keep you relaxed.

Some Hints for Relaxation at Work

- If you work with a VDU, telephone operating machine, typewriter, photocopier, or conveyor belt, or operate machinery with repetitive movements, make sure you take regular breaks (five minutes every hour if possible).

- To release tension in the shoulders and neck, raise your shoulders up to your ears, tense the muscles, then drop them; repeat this nine more times.

- Every hour take a few minutes to stretch. Put your arms above your head, palms together, link your fingers, turn palms outwards, stretch upwards and hold for the count of 20.

- Rotate your wrists, five times to the left, then five times to the right.

- Stand up, feet apart, knees bent, your weight over your knees (watch your lower back doesn't bend inwards too far because you could do yourself damage) and let your arms swing loose while you let your head drop. Hold this position for a count of 20.

- Stand up, drop your chin on your chest, then turn your head to the left, let your head roll back while you look up at the ceiling, then roll it round to the right and back to chin on your chest. Do this slowly five times. Then go the other way.

- Still standing, open your arms out to the side, palms down, then bring the hands back to meet across the chest, then spread your arms out again. Do this five times, to open your chest after hunching.

- Finally, open your mouth as wide as you can, stretching your jaw and cheek muscles, then relax. Do this five times. Let yourself yawn and yawn. You can start yourself yawning by wiggling your jaw side to side and opening your mouth wide (yawning is a profoundly healing form of physical tension release).

Of course, you don't have to do these exercises all at once. Do one or two every so often. But keep moving and loose, and try and keep relaxed.

Try to avoid alcohol at work (especially important in occupations where industrial injuries are a potential hazard, and if you're driving home), because it's tiring. Try not to call at the pub on the way home, or walk in the door and pour a gin and tonic. Give yourself half an hour of 'quiet' time, if possible. I know this is very hard if you have children and/or your partner also works, or you're a single parent, but try.

A Simple Meditation Technique

This is like the simple relaxation technique, but whereas that was about relaxing the body primarily, this one is about relaxing the mind. Of course, as the mind and body are linked, these two techniques complement each other.

Set aside at least 15 minutes both morning and evening. The more time you allocate to meditation, the greater the rewards. Meditation is about stilling the mind, calming you down, so you can just 'sit' and 'be'. It is a profound contradiction to the hassle and hustle of everyday life.

Again use a timer or alarm clock to set your time. You need to be quiet and undisturbed, so try and be in a room on your own, with no phone interruptions. Lock the door (if possible).

- Sit upright in a crossed-legged fashion, if you can. If not, get comfortable with your back upright supported against a wall, and with your feet straight out in front, or brought up together in a semi-cross-legged position.

- Place your hands on your thighs, or let them flop by your side. Close your eyes, and simply concentrate on your breathing. As you breathe in, think 'rising' and as you breathe out, think 'falling'. That is all you have to do – over and over and over.

At first it may seem strange or awkward, but let yourself continue to think 'rising' and 'falling' in time with your breaths. You will probably find your mind whizzing around, worries popping out, plans hatching – but keep bringing your mind back to the words. Don't wriggle, or scratch, or move. If you feel an itch, ignore it and concentrate on the words. Just keep on coming back to centre. After a while you will enter what is called the 'Alpha State', where your brain waves slow down and you become deeply relaxed. You will feel very focused on your breathing, very still and almost floating in time.

When your timer goes off   – don't jump up and back to life immediately. Take your time.

During the day, you can use train journeys, or when waiting for people, or for meetings, as times to meditate. You could use 10 minutes of your lunch break or perhaps your tea break. And last thing at night, half an hour, or even 15 minutes, will be very beneficial, enabling you to become peaceful enough to go to sleep.

- Solitude. A lot of us are frightened of solitude, but it is a definite need. Find some time to 'be alone', if you can, each day. It may be going for a walk, gardening, knitting or reading a book. You may well need to organize time to be alone by being very straight with people you live with. This can be very difficult, especially for women who are 'on duty' to meet everyone's needs all the time. But even a long hot bath can be used as a way to get some space.

SLEEP

Sleep is the great healer, allowing the body to repair itself and the mind to sift through experiences in the form of dreams. Some people fall asleep as their heads hit the pillow, while others toss and turn for hours. The more you worry about sleep, the less relaxed you'll be about sleeping.

To get your physical needs met for sleep, you might need to experiment. Do you, for instance, respond well to naps in the middle of the day? Do you need to sleep in total darkness? Do you need ear-plugs for total silence?

How many hours sleep do you need on average? People generally need less sleep as they age, but we vary greatly. Also, going through emotional upheavals, such as bereavement, moving house, changing your job, or being in therapy, will probably make you feel tired. Sometimes you can feel exhausted even though you have had a 'good night's sleep' of 12 or 13 hours and at other times you can feel refreshed after four.

Some Helpful Hints on Sleep

- Alcohol, caffeine and other mind-changing drugs actually disturb your sleep, so having an alcoholic 'nightcap' might have the opposite effect to what you want. If you go to bed having drunk alcohol, also drink at least a pint of water, to prevent dehydration. Other times, drink warm milk with a dash of honey; or herb teas such as camomile or special bedtime mixtures, are relaxing.

- Wind down if you work late; don't go straight from staring at a word processor screen or being on night duty to bed.

Give yourself time to relax. Have a bath, meditate, read a book, or listen to some soothing music.

- Avoid eating late, which is heavy on your digestive system and may give you disturbed sleep, even nightmares.

- Write a diary. This is a very therapeutic way of ending your day, where you can empty out your thoughts, feelings and frustrations.

- Talk into a cassette recorder, or even to the cat, as if you are talking to a good friend.

- Release some emotions – maybe cry, or yawn, talk on the phone to someone about what's bothering you. Get feelings 'off your chest'.

- Make a list of what you have to do next day. Sometimes you go to bed and your mind is churning; you are worried that you won't remember everything you need to do, so it's a good idea to jot it all down. Keep paper and pen by the bed so that if you wake in the night, thinking about what you've got to do, again, you can make a list and then go back to sleep.

- Relax in bed. Follow the simple relaxation technique described on pages 192–3.

- Masturbate/have sex. A lot of people do this to get to sleep. It can also be used as a way of relieving tension, although beware of getting into an addictive ritual about having to do it every night.

- Burn some relaxing aromatherapy oils, such as sandalwood and rosemary in your room before you go to sleep.

- Make sure the room is ventilated; fresh air is important.

- Make sure your bed is comfortable. Many people put up with the most appalling beds, so check yours is well-sprung, but firm and supporting your back properly. If you are allergic to feathers, change to hollofil pillows and duvet, and only use synthetic blankets and bed covers. Make sure you have got enough space if there are two of you in bed and that the bed doesn't sag in the middle. Beds are worth spending money on, given how much time we spend in them.

- Try to ensure that your bedroom is in a quiet place in your home; if this is difficult, buy some earplugs and use them.

- Get massaged. If you have a willing partner, ask him or her to massage you with some oil or body lotion. Touch is a great healer and relaxer and will help you to sleep more peacefully.

Be Powerful About Your Sleep Needs

Think about how much sleep you need and try to get it. Research shows that if you sleep lots at weekends it can throw your biorhythms out, so the idea of 'catching up' on sleep can be somewhat misleading. Often it is the psychological and emotional impact of not sleeping that causes more of a problem than the physiology. Humans are pretty resilient and parents lose masses of sleep while rearing children. It's not ideal, but they survive. The most important thing is to know what you need and be powerful about getting it.

Sleep and Relationships

Different sleep patterns and needs can be a bone of contention in relationships – where one partner's needs dictate how the other should sleep. Roughly, people divide into 'owls', who tend to stay up late, and find it hard to get up in the morning; and 'larks' who wake up early and get up easily, but start crashing out any time after 10 pm. Relationships between owls and larks can be problematic.

The solution?

- Talk about it. Often, simply airing the differences will relieve some tension. Take turns listening to each other, really try to understand the other person's perspective.

- Compromise. If one of you must have the light off at 11 pm and the other wants to read, you could fix up a light that beams only on to the reader's book, without disturbing the sleeper. Or you could sleep separately. Or the reader could read elsewhere, and then come quietly to bed. Or the sleeper could wear an eye mask to keep the light out (you could take it in turns as to who does what).

- Accept that everyone is different and has their own foibles. What you do isn't the ultimate measure of what is right. Equally, you don't have to accept what your partner does as the rule of thumb. Keep talking, negotiating, compromising – and you should both get your physical needs met amicably.

Chapter 12

———o———

Meeting Your Sexual Needs

Sex involves all sorts of needs: emotional, physical, intellectual and spiritual. Sex can be the most wonderful, uplifting experience; it can also be unsatisfying, boring, even frightening. Sex can be very confusing – conflicting messages surround us all the time on billboards, TV, in films and magazines. Not understanding your sexual needs and how to meet them healthily can lead to a lot of misery, which in turn can lead you to suppressing your feelings through chemical and emotional addictions.

You might be waiting for the 'perfect sexual partner' to appear, someone who will satisfy your every need, without you saying a word. This is fantasy. And it leaves you powerless and dissatisfied. Yet, having a good, healthy and safe sex life is the concern of millions, if the letters to 'Agony Aunts', and the popular radio and TV phone-ins are any guide. Although we are now much more open about having sex before, during and outside marriage, sex is still discussed almost incessantly in the media because many people (especially women) find good sex elusive. The experience of sex remains intensely personal and each person's sexual needs are unique.

LOVE AND SEX

Of course, you can have love without sex, and sex without love. People always have, although we've only really started being open about it over the past thirty years. Once we become sexually active in our teens and twenties, we usually try out several, or many partners, with or without falling in love. Getting it right can take some time to learn. But it is most important that you do know what you want sexually; and you may only find out through experimentation and forming different sorts of sexual relationships.

Reproduction

Looked at coldly, sex is purely a means for the human race to reproduce itself. Indeed, some people feel this 'biological drive' is the primary force behind forming sexual relationships, and may only have sex when they want to reproduce, due to religious, cultural or personal beliefs. But with the introduction of modern reproductive technology, such as In Vitro Fertilization (IVF) it is now possible to reproduce human beings from a test tube, without sexual intercourse taking place at all.

Sexual Preference

Sexual preference also affects the purpose of sex. Because gay men, lesbian women and bisexuals have sexual relationships with their own gender, this obviously makes reproduction with each other impossible. However, some gay men and lesbians have got round this problem by adopting or fostering children, being parents to their partners' offspring from previous heterosexual relationships, using IVF, or surrogacy (where a woman carries and gives birth to a child for another person or couple). So your biology doesn't necessarily dictate your destiny any more.

AIDS

Since AIDS became world news, we have all had to examine our sexual behaviour afresh. Today, our sexual needs must necessarily be tempered by having 'Safe Sex', which has meant having to be honest with ourselves, and others about our sexual habits, preferences and partners. At one time, gay men were believed to be the sole carriers of AIDS. We now know this is not true, and that the whole population needs to practise safe sex. No one is immune from AIDS.

Sexual Addiction

Sexual addiction has begun to be recognized as a serious issue for people who feel the only time they are really alive, loved and connected is when they are having sex (and/or conquering another sexual partner). This is when sex is used to try to meet those frozen needs for love, affection, validation and care which were never met in the past, and which can never be compensated for in the present. If someone is sexually addicted, they usually need to face the feelings (usually isolation and low self-esteem) which emerge when they are not sexually active. Then real needs for love, affection, acceptance need to be met. An extreme form of sexual addiction is sado-masochism, where one partner dominates another by inflicting pain and humiliation.

Pornography

Pornography can stimulate sexual addiction, too. It seems to offer unlimited, unreal sex with celluoid images to (mainly) men and some women. In a sense, these images offer to meet their frozen needs for total acceptance, instant sexual gratification and endless pleasure, without having to relate to an actual partner. Of course, pornography is often the only sex education that men get. But it can provide a fairly repetitive and degrading stimulus to masturbate over, and can lead to disappointment, confusion and penis-centred sexual attitudes in real life.

Sexual Fantasies

Pornography also fuels sexual fantasies – which in themselves may be banal – but when applied to life can be disturbing, even dangerous, especially if someone wants to act them out *without* their partner's consent. Sexual fantasies can also distance people from each other emotionally. So although fantasies can be powerfully exciting, they can be addictive, making it harder for people to relate to each other sexually in the present. Although many books on sex suggest couples fantasize to 'come' with each other, this can be emotionally dishonest in a loving, sexual relationship. You can get so focused on reaching orgasm that you forget you are in bed with a person, with whom you are having a relationship, as you fantasize about making love to a film star or ex-lover in your head. This can mean losing out on real, loving intimacy and sexual pleasure. If your sex life together isn't very inspiring then it is far healthier to talk about how it might be improved, rather than continue to pretend. You will get closer and respect each other more. It can be a great relief to get things out in the open because there can be so much secret fear about 'performance' attached to sex.

Sexual Self-Esteem

This pressure to 'prove' yourself sexually is especially tough on men. And there is also a lot of pressure to 'attract' people sexually if you're a woman (although men are becoming increasingly concerned about how they measure up to current ideas of the body beautiful). Some people will go to great lengths (and great pains) to make themselves ever more desir-able, via plastic surgery and implants to faces, breasts, thighs, penises, and even chest hair.

Regardless of the skill of any surgeon's scalpel, the real issue is how you feel inside about your own sexuality (and body), and how well you know your own sexual needs. Your self-esteem won't really grow from keeping score of your sexual conquests or having enormous pectorals and/or breasts. It *will* develop more healthily from simply liking, loving and accepting yourself.

How to Improve Your Sexual Self-Esteem

- Accept your body for what it is, how it looks, its uniqueness. You can't be perfect, nobody is. Spend time looking at yourself in a mirror. Look at the parts of your body you like. Look at your own genitals in a mirror – examine their beauty, their symmetry, get accustomed to your body and how it looks and works – it's wonderful.

- Make the best of yourself by meeting your physical needs (see Chapter 11), especially for diet and nutrition, exercise and fitness, relaxation and sleep. Good food, regular exercise and rest will tone you up and make you feel much better about yourself. Treat your body well – you deserve it.

- Make a list of what is attractive about you. Don't be shy and don't just think, 'nothing'. What about your hair or skin colour, your character (lively, friendly, kind, fun-loving) etcetera? Blow your own trumpet – to yourself anyway.

- If you have been sexually active in the past (or are currently), think about sexual experiences you have had where you have felt you were an attentive and thoughtful lover, where you have been close and tender with another person, where you have had fun. And think about pleasure you have given to someone (rather than just taken). Good sex isn't just down to technique (although that matters to some extent). It is more about feeling, about being playful and sensual, about communicating while loving. Of course, sex can be fierce and passionate, it can also be tender and gentle.

So what makes you a good lover? Write down in your notebook whatever comes to mind. But answer the question honestly. Don't fantasize.

....
....

Also, can you remember a time when someone made you feel
loved and cared for sexually? What made them a good lover
for you? Write it down to help highlight your needs.

....

....

KNOWING YOUR OWN SEXUAL
NEEDS

Our sexuality is ever developing, although we're usually led to
believe that we have a fixed 'sexual identity' for life. Not so. All
sorts of circumstances can change who you relate to sexually.
Think of your sexuality and your sex life as a railway track
along which there are different stations. You begin chugging
along at puberty and then you stop at different stations as you
progress though life. Sometimes you may be sexually inactive
either through choice or circumstance. Sometimes you may be
highly sexually active. Eventually you might have a steady
(safe, but a bit mundane) sex life with one person, perhaps for
years (even for life). Or, you might be heterosexual, bisexual,
gay or lesbian at different times, too, stopping at other stations
down the line.

Perhaps your major sexual relationship is with yourself,
through masturbation, and this suits you fine. Or maybe you
are satisfied with your regular partner because you feel loved
and cared for. Whatever the case for you, it's important to get
to know your own sexual needs. Why? Because it will improve
your sexual relationship(s) no end if you can be clear about
your particular needs.

At the same time, you might feel unhappy about your
sexuality. For instance, you might fear you are gay when you
are in fact, a married man with children. This is not uncom-
mon, yet it can create a lot of emotional pain because of the
fear of not being 'normal'. You might need to talk to a good
friend, a counsellor, the Samaritans, your doctor, or a specialist agency, like Gay Switchboard, about how you feel (see
'Help' section). You may need to look at your own sexual

history, at your emotional needs and try to work out what you want for yourself. Most important of all is to accept yourself for what you are, no matter how confused or frightened you may feel. You might need to be able to face and release your feelings about your sexuality – if this is true for you, go back to Chapter 10: Meeting Your Emotional Needs and remind yourself how.

No Coercion

Whatever form your sex life takes, never coerce anyone else into doing something they don't want to do, or allow yourself to be so coerced. Of course, sometimes you don't know whether you will like something or not until you have tried it. But if you sense instinctively that you don't want to be tied up with ropes or beaten with a riding crop in a sado-masochistic fantasy, then don't let anyone do that to you. Be aware of your rights, and of other people's. You may well be trying to meet particular emotional needs through sex, such as anger or taking revenge. Certainly, young people should never, ever be coerced by you or anyone else, to be sexual.

Communication

Communication between partners is essential for meeting your sexual needs. Open your notebook again as you ask yourself right now (if you're in a sexual relationship):

1. Are you totally satisfied with your sex life?

....

If not, what needs to change?

....

2. What is stopping you from being direct about what you need or want from your partner(s)?

....

3. What do you need to communicate about your sexual needs?

....

If you are not communicating about sex and yet you are dissatisfied, then there may be something going awry in your relationship at a deeper level. Your sex life going off the boil is often one of the first signs that a relationship is in trouble. At the same time, work stress, money problems, pregnancy, illness and other issues can contribute to a disrupted sex life. Talking about sex can be really explosive, because it can touch raw nerves about your sexual self-esteem, but is essential if you want to keep channels of communication open.

If you feel there is something that needs saying, why not:

- Suggest that you and your partner sit down together to talk about sex (you can say there is something you need to talk about, but you find it difficult to say).

- Say what is bothering you in an unattacking way. Don't just launch into, 'you always roll on and off, and start snoring within three minutes, you selfish pig'. Say, 'I'm not finding our sex life very satisfying at present. I'd like to talk about how we could both improve it.' (You could even write a letter to get your thoughts straight, although it is better to talk face to face.) Whether your partner is aware or not that something is wrong, he or she will usually want to improve your mutual sexual pleasure – so that is a tactful way in.

- If it is your partner who initiates such a talk, try to listen without jumping in and defending yourself. It may feel very hard to take what the other person is saying to you because it can feel like a personal attack – but remember they're trying to tell you something that matters to them and which they find very hard to say.

- Agree a course of action. It is a good idea, if sex is not working, to abstain for a while and simply cuddle and get close instead. Start talking about what you like about each other. Just getting into the usual sexual routine can mean you bypass how you are really feeling. You could massage each other, having agreed beforehand not to be sexual, to relieve any pressure to perform. Enjoy and explore each other's bodies. Sex isn't just about orgasm, it is about connecting with another person (and yourself) lovingly, and giving and receiving pleasure. If you have both got into a rut, just focus on having physical pleasure without sex while continuing to talk.

• You might consider having sex therapy as a couple. Relate, the national counselling agency for couples, can advise. To talk about your sex life in confidence with an impartial third party can often help. It may not be easy to say things at first, but it can ease communication long-term. (See 'Help' section.)

Single, and/or Celibate

You need to think carefully about how to meet your own sexual needs.

• You might choose to be celibate. Some people believe they save precious energy by not having sexual relationships with other people, or even masturbating to orgasm. Certainly, some people feel a heightened spiritual, intellectual and/or creative awareness, and experience increased productivity at work when celibate. Don't let anyone make you feel bad about being celibate. It can be a very positive, healing choice, especially if you are recovering from the end of an important sexual relationship, the death of a partner or even sexual abuse.

• You may masturbate. Be aware of your sexual needs, which for women might mean heightened sexual feelings around their time of menstruation, due to changes in hormone levels. Some people may need to masturbate every night, others two or three times a week. Whatever your need, as you make love to yourself, care about your body. Some people (especially men) can get addicted to masturbation as a form of sleeping pill or comforter when lonely, and feel hollow, sordid and lonely afterwards. If you are masturbating in that way, then it could be a good idea to talk to

someone in confidence about it. There is nothing wrong
with you, but the negative feelings that come after masturbating are an indication that your real emotional needs are
not being met. If you can focus on meeting these needs,
then your sex life may well improve. Whatever you do, don't
damage yourself by inserting dangerous or sharp objects
into your body or inflicting self-mutilation. You are worth
more than this kind of self-abuse.

AND FINALLY . . .

If you are sexually active, whatever your age, sexual preference and particular circumstance, practise safe sex:

- Take time to talk to and get to know your lover.

- Don't assume a virtual stranger is 'safe' because he or she is
  'nice'.

- Be imaginative – experiment.

- Only have sex if you want to, and you both want it.

- If it doesn't feel good – don't do it.

- Always use a condom and a water-based lubricant.

Meet your own sexual needs by being sensuous, sensitive and
sensible.

Chapter 13

———◦———

Meeting Your Social Needs

Human beings are social animals, with a real need to get close to, connect and communicate with each other. Social interaction happens in all sorts of ways – in the formal relationships you have at work, or with people who provide professional services, such as builders and solicitors; and in the informal relationships you have through love and sexual relationships, family networks and friendships.

Yet, even though we are often surrounded by people in social settings, we can experience intense isolation. Because our society is so highly industrialized, most of us live in cities today, or in large urban and suburban sprawls. The decline of rural life has meant communities have dwindled, with many young people and families migrating to large towns and cities to find work. What were well-established country communities are now often largely populated with commuting executives, or urban dwellers seeking an idyllic pastoral weekend life. At the same time, families have become smaller, and single parent families are on the increase with one in two marriages collapsing. So the old system of extended family is becoming rare, and loneliness is on the increase.

ISOLATION AS A TRIGGER FOR ADDICTION

If you feel isolated in the middle of a large city or town, it can seem daunting to have to 'break into' existing networks to create a social life. Conversely, if you are an urbanite, heading for the country, the local town or village may not yield to your charms as quickly as you hope. You can feel very alone wherever you are, whatever you are doing and whatever your circumstances. When you feel lonely, that nobody cares or loves you, that it's up to you to do everything for yourself, you can feel in great need of comfort. And that is where addictions come in, as we saw in Part 1 of this book.

No Substitute

Addictions are no substitute for real social contact. Although they are often used as a means of bringing people together and lowering inhibitions (particularly alcohol at parties and get-togethers), they can become an end in themselves. Of course, glue-sniffers will congregate with glue-sniffers, and wine-tasters with wine-tasters, but the real need for meaningful contact can get lost. When people meet around an addiction, they are relating to the addictive behaviour rather than to the people involved.

You can be wildly high on dope at a party, but still feel achingly lonely within. You can be having outrageously exciting sex with someone, and still feel unloved and alone. You can be the best employee at work, getting all the accolades for performance, and be totally isolated in your workaholism. You can be an exemplary mother in the Women's Institute, and still feel nobody understands your private struggles and sorrows.

Few of us get time to sit back and think about our social needs. Maybe it's a visit to the pub after work? Or maybe it is meeting with mothers and toddlers in your village hall? Perhaps you find it easy to start chatting to people at the bus stop or at your evening class. Or do you feel you have no need of other people, and watch TV most of the time? Whatever you do or don't do, you may well have a nagging feeling, somewhere deep down, that you are missing out. That other people are having a rip-roaring social life, out every night, meeting fascinating people, and feeling fully satisfied. You may feel envious of people you know who don't seem to have to 'do' anything, yet always have friends dropping in for a cuppa or supper. We can all feel that someone, somewhere else, is having a better time than we are.

The most important thing to note about your social needs is that you have them. It is entirely 'natural' to want to go out and meet people. If you feel daunted by the prospect, then it could be your own isolation and fear that is getting in the way. But you don't have to disappear under these feelings. You just have to acknowledge them and decide to push past them if you want your social needs to be met.

What Are Your Social Needs?

Before we go any further, let's look at what your own social needs are. Answer the following questions in your notebook.

1. What is your social life like right now? What do you do with other people socially? What activities do you enjoy?
    ....

2. Are you satisfied with your social life? If not, how would you like it to change?
    ....

3. What, if anything, is stopping you from getting your social needs met?
    ....

4. If you could prioritize one area of your social life that you would like to change, what would it be?
    ....

5. What do you need to do? What is your first step?
    ....

Your Self-Esteem

Your self-esteem bears a direct relationship to how well your social needs are being met. As we've already seen in Chapter 9, you can build your self-esteem by deciding to be your own parent and give yourself what you need. Once you get into the swing of believing you deserve improved social relationships, your self-esteem will then begin to flower. You can nourish your self-esteem by nourishing your social needs.

Your Relationships

Because addictions are based on feeling lonely, isolated, unlovable, disconnected, and unworthy, one of the most powerful ways you can get off the hook is to decide to meet your own social needs. With this in mind, the following are general 'tips' which you will need to adapt to your own particular situation.

To start with, you need to look at your present social relationships. The drawing below represents you at the centre – the concentric circles represent levels of intimacy and closeness. Copy this drawing into your notebook and put yourself at the centre. Then put in the names of people in your life, with the closest nearest you, the least close the farthest away.

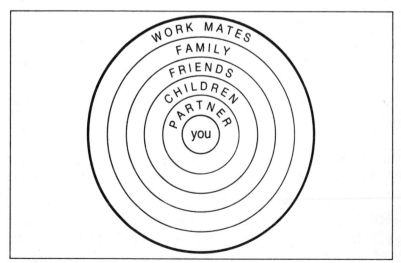

This should give you a picture of your social relationships as they currently exist. That is, whom you can rely on, who you feel is 'there' for you, whom you love.

Ask yourself, and write down the answers in your notebook:

1. How much do you trust each one?

   ....

2. Have you got into a rut or are your relationships moving forward?

   ....

3. Who takes the initiative? Who makes contact? Who organizes things you do together?

   ....

4. Are they equal, mutually satisfying relationships or generally one-sided?

   ....

Meeting Your Own Social Needs

Roughly, social needs are the need for:

- Communication. Conversation (including small talk), exchange of information and ideas, discussion and debate.

- Love and validation. Feeling worthwhile, cared for, valued.

- A sense of belonging. This can be to your family, community, neighbourhood, at work, to specialist groups and organizations, to your village, town or city, to your social group.

- Meaningful activities. These may include charity work, beautifying your garden and house, working for a worthwhile cause, caring for people.

Here are some suggestions for ways in which you can meet all of those social needs. See which ones most appeal to you and start with them.

Give up waiting. Your social needs will not be met by magic. As with other needs, you have to decide to meet them for yourself. If you remain passive about your social life and bitter and envious about other people's good fortune, you are acting powerlessly. Give up waiting for someone else to make the first move. You can take charge, right now.

Take the initiative. Pick up the phone and call someone and/or talk to someone at work. It may seem scary the first few times, but it will get easier as you practice. If you want to see a film with a particular person, ask them. Assume they will be delighted to go with you, that you are a fine person to spend time with.

Don't try too hard. You don't need to convince anyone that you're brilliant, fun to be with, exciting, brave, talented or monied. When you are with people, whether at work, at home, on the street, or at a party, relax. Assume they will like you and that you don't need to convince them you are likeable. Often we try too hard to impress, to make things happen. Relax and let things evolve. Don't force the situation into what you want it to be. That is being too controlling and people shy away from feeling manipulated and dominated.

Listen well. People love being listened to. There are very few people who listen well. We are nearly always preparing our next statement, argument or fact while someone else is talking. Good listeners are always popular because they bring people out of themselves, they make people feel safe and none of us has been listened to enough, so being with you can be a treat.

Take your turn to speak. On the other hand, people don't feel comfortable with someone who never reveals anything about themselves. If you only ever listen, you never spill the beans, you are never vulnerable, other people will feel that you don't trust them. They may feel rejected, or that you are stand-offish, or that you don't like them. Give them a chance to listen to you.

Be real.   We often pretend because we feel uncertain of ourselves. If you are trembling with fear when you meet someone new – say on a date – you can admit, very lightly, to being a bit shy or embarrassed. People usually warm to you if you admit the truth. This does not mean going into a major diatribe about your terrible childhood on the first meeting, and scaring someone off. It means be real, don't pretend, be yourself; but be conscious that another person is involved.

Be realistic.   You might have a fantasy about how a party, a wedding, or an office get-together will be. That is fine – vision is essential for making things happen socially. But don't be unrealistic about what you can achieve at one event, because you will inevitably be disappointed and then feel discouraged about doing something like that again. Have realistic expectations about what you can achieve socially.

Be thoughtful.   If you are inviting people from different backgrounds, religions, cultures to meet together, be thoughtful about them. For instance, don't ask Jewish people to come to supper on Friday night, as this is Shabbas. Be appropriate with your suggestions.

Don't give up.   Some people will try something only once and then give up because it did not work instantly. It can take many different approaches to make something work. Experiment. Put different people together and see how they mix. It can take time to work out what a successful formula is for a dinner party or works outing.

Meeting New People

Meeting new people can be a nightmare for anyone who feels painfully shy or awkward in social situations. Really, there's no short-cut to just doing it, doing it, doing it until you feel more comfortable. And you *will* feel more comfortable once your social network starts growing. Here are some tips for meeting new people:

Try new things.   Join an evening class, take up a new sport, go to a restaurant you haven't been to before, join a network based on a particular interest or activity, like 1930's films or chess.

Strike up conversations.   This can feel very scary, but if you read a daily newspaper, or are at an event such as an exhibition or summer sale, or you are at your local swimming pool – chat to people. It does not have to be deeply meaningful, nor should it be a one-sided moan. That seldom wins you friends. If you can be humorous and light with people, they will be cheered up by your positive energy.

Join a reputable dating agency – or advertise in newspapers or journals (using a box number). This way, you can meet people with similar interests if you are shy. If you advertise and ask for a photo of the other person, then you have power in your hands. If you meet someone you like, but don't fancy, you can set up a monthly dinner at a restaurant where you each bring a different same gender friend each month. If you are a man, you bring a male friend; if you are a woman, you bring a female friend. This is a good way to extend your friendship network, and with any luck you may fancy each others' friends as well. Of course, you need to protect yourself as you would on any date – don't give your address and phone number out unless you want to, and don't get pressurized into sexual contact.

Keep your eyes open.   For like-minded people at work, people who make you laugh at your evening class, friendly women at your local women's centre, and interesting people in your street. Once you start looking, you will find a wide range of people you can relate to. And they have friends, brothers, colleagues, families – in time you might meet them too.

Be open-minded.   It is very easy to dismiss people on first acquaintance. We make so many assumptions about accents, class, clothes, skin colour, age and physical ability. Suspend your prejudices and really look to see the person underneath.

Give someone time to open up with you before you pass judgement – don't just write them off after one meeting. You may well be wrong. It takes time to really get to know people, and they will probably surprise you.

Meeting People at Work

If you work, you probably spend a lot of time either there, or commuting back and forth. Maybe you are the kind of person who likes to 'keep themselves to themselves', and work is just a place to earn money. Or maybe you throw yourself into your work, and always form relationships and friendships with people you work with. Whatever, work can meet your social needs:

- If you feel your work is meaningful and you are committed to it, it will meet a very deep need for making a worthwhile contribution. If you spend your life, say, making the little paper umbrellas that decorate cocktail drinks, it is very hard to feel you're making a real contribution, and this in turn will affect your self-esteem. But even if you *are* making cocktail umbrellas, you can babysit for someone, or dig an older person's garden, or buy groceries for someone who is sick. This kind of activity isn't one-way giving to the other person either, it actually feeds a deep need in yourself for connection, for doing something meaningful.

- Suggest social events. This could be an office party or works outing, a monthly women's meeting, a monthly lunch. Or you might play squash or go swimming with someone after work. Be thoughtful about your relationships at work, however. Don't force yourself on to people who don't want to be sociable, or have too many other commitments. This can lead to people feeling sexually harassed or pressurized. Also keep a sense of what is appropriate. Don't go up to the managing director and invite him or her to go out to lunch with you. Be aware of your formal roles and how socializing can affect them.

- Don't gossip. If someone at work reveals something personal to you – that they have had an abortion, or their wife has left them, keep it to yourself. Respect the confidence and show you are worthy of it. You may be bursting to tell someone but gossip breeds gossip, and can get very distorted as it gets passed on. In the end you will just be known as the big-mouth who can't be trusted. And although people may rush to you to get the latest, they won't really want to be your friend.

- Be private. Sometimes you may be dying to tell someone your tragic or wonderful news, but this may not be appropriate and may be used against you. If it is serious personal news, such as a death in the family, tell your personnel officer, your boss and/or a close colleague. If you start a sexual relationship with someone at work, it is probably a very good idea to keep it private; otherwise you may jeopardize both your positions. Confide only in those people you know to be trustworthy either because of their position in relation to you, or because you know them well.

Social Life

Your social life can take many forms, from simply having people round for a meal or going out to dinner, to being involved in particular activities, such as Go-Karting or Green Party politics.

Apart from all the general points above, there are some specific tips, particularly about entertaining:

Being entertained. Don't be a pain. If you are invited to someone's house for a meal, make sure you arrive on time and that you bring something with you, say a bunch of flowers, or a bottle of wine or mineral water. If the invitation is just for a cup of tea, then you could bring biscuits or fruit. A small gesture is often appreciated.

If you have particular dietary requirements and you are asked for dinner – take the initiative and explain your needs at the time the invitation is received. Offer to bring something yourself. So, if you're vegan, for instance, say you will bring soya milk and extra fruit and salad. If you don't drink alcohol, bring something non-alcoholic with you as your contribution.

But don't make your particular beliefs about food your main topic of conversation.

Don't embarrass your host or put other people down by airing a morally superior viewpoint. This is extremely off-putting. If someone else wants to eat chocolate, that is up to them. It is not up to you to lecture them. It certainly won't win you new friends or a great social life, because clearly you can only interact with people in a similar narrow vein to yourself.

Finally, be courteous. Thank your host for the meal, cup of tea, a short visit, or whatever. Offer to wash up or buy food if you stay for several days. Send a card saying 'thank you' after staying the night or a weekend. It makes people feel their efforts are appreciated, and they are more likely to invite you again.

Entertaining. If you are inviting someone for a meal or to stay over, ask them if they have particular needs. For instance, they may be allergic to feather pillows, or can't drink coffee. If you know ahead of time who is vegetarian, your dinner party menu can be tailor-made. There is nothing worse than someone arriving and not being able to enjoy the results of your hours of effort in the kitchen. Make sure that you treat such guests with relaxed courtesy. There is nothing so tense-making as an over-elaborate meal, with the host over-dressed, red in the face and too exhausted to enjoy the occasion. If you can strike a balance and be casually organized, then people will want to invite you back.

We're often lax about asking people what they want. For all you know, your weekend guest would like to relax and sit in the garden, rather than be hauled round the local shops and sites of interest. Just ask and listen, then organize matters to suit you, your family and your guest(s). If you haven't much money but like to entertain, you could ask guests to bring one dish each, to share. You may think this is a bit of a cheek, but people are usually very willing to bring something, like a starter or a pudding, and they actually feel more involved in the meal because they have made a contribution. It costs you less and involves them more – and can be a good way to make friends.

Parties

Few of us organize parties without food, drinks and possibly drugs, forming the focal point. That may be what you have always done, and what you think people want. Yet, there are so many other ways in which people can be sociable with each other, *and* get off the hook of addictions.

If you think organized activities are central to enjoyment, then there are all sorts of ways in which you can make parties less addiction-focused.

Treasure hunts.   You can organize a treasure hunt in a local park, your garden, around your neighbourhood. The prize should be back at your place. Send out invitations (a photo-copied piece of A4 is fine) so that people know the kind of party you're going to have. When guests arrive, suggest they go in pairs (not in their partnerships), so they can get to know someone new.

Picnics.   Suggest you meet at a certain spot in a local park or garden, and all bring a dish and a bottle. Have plenty of non-alcoholic drinks and fresh fruit available, so there are alternatives to alcohol and junk food.

Party games.   Have an adults' party with party games – anything from blowing bubbles, water pistols, balloons, board games, like Trivial Pursuit, or physical board games, like Twister. You may think 'aaagh' not in my house – but games of all sorts are great ice-breakers and you can have lots of fun. Certainly more than you can when just holding a glass of plonk and standing around trying to keep the conversation going. Most people know how to play pass the parcel, stick the tail on the donkey and 'consequences', and as the party warms up any initial slight embarrassment will soon be forgotten.

Celebrate Halloween, Bonfire Night, Christmas, etc.   You can dress up, use face paints, play charades, have a cabaret, sing songs (you can have song sheets for people who don't know the words).

Brunches. If you feel daunted by inviting people to meals and parties and feel it would be too alcohol/addiction-centred, invite people round for Sunday brunch. This is a combined breakfast and lunch. Invite four to six guests and serve breakfast foods, like croissants, muesli, bread, honey, cheese, yoghurt and fruit. You don't have to serve alcohol; provide decaffeinated tea and coffee and fruit juices. And get in three or four of the Sunday papers. This can be a very relaxed event which doesn't put too much stress on anybody, and enables social relationships to grow.

DO WHAT YOU WANT, NOT WHAT YOU OUGHT

You might think some of the above suggestions are not 'you', or even that you would be too embarrassed to try any of them. Or maybe you have always secretly wanted to have an adult's play party, but feel other people would think you are silly. If you operate from what you want to do, rather than what you think you ought to do, you will be a social hit with people because the event will emanate from your passion, sense of fun and enjoyment, rather than from duty.

If you love dancing to music, invite friends to dance with you. If you love swimming, have a swimming party. If you love old movies, invite a group round to watch one with you.

Being sociable doesn't have to be either expensive or difficult. It is all about you deciding to meet your social needs, to stop being isolated, and to connect with other human beings through particular activities and events. If you feel you can have fun and be close to people without chemical and emotional addictions being involved, you will be meeting your *real* social needs instead.

Chapter 14

———○———

Meeting Your Creative Needs

The word 'creative' can be off-putting, conjuring up images of pretentious people saying 'dahling' to each other in loud voices. This is, of course, a caricature. As a culture we depend on other people's creativity to entertain us, lift our spirits, enrich our souls, beautify our environment, fill us with vision, create our furniture, cars and clothes. In fact, we *all* have immense amounts of untapped creative energy which can be opened up, channelled and developed. A crucial part of overcoming addiction is being able to identify and nurture your own creative needs. Any creative activity will nourish your soul, spirit and self. Being creative is a way of bringing together everything you know about yourself and your world. Your creativity is a blend of all of your skills, perceptions, ideas, experiences – indeed, it is *you*.

'SHOWING OFF'

A regular feature of my residential addictions workshops are playing games, singing songs and having a Saturday night 'Cabaret'. This has evolved over the years. I ask people to bring all sorts of 'props' with them: dressing up clothes, party clothes, glitter sprays, make-up, face paints, favourite dance cassettes and anything they'd like to 'show off'. This part of the workshop usually brings shrieks of embarrassed laughter and much shivering with fear. Some people want to run away and hide, remembering awful times of public humiliation at school, at home, with friends. But by the end of the 'showing off' time *everyone* has usually had a great time.

First of all, everyone has 10 minutes to think about what they want to 'show off' about themselves, and then people take it in turns in front of the group. The group's job is to provide a warm, appreciative audience – not to heckle and look bored. Shy, embarrassed or proud, 'performers' tremble and blush as they sing a song, show-off their legs, pass round a piece of jewellery or pottery that they've made, or display a jumper they've hand-knitted, or even recite a poem. Nearly everyone feels awkward and braces themselves for attack and criticism. So when they get wholehearted applause, you can see their self-esteem soaring.

I then get people into small groups of four or five and they go off and work out a song or sketch to do in front of the group. Half an hour is ample time and people come up with all sorts of ingenious things – rewriting popular songs, producing original songs with musical accompaniment, complete one-act plays, and abstract dances. You can see people grow in confidence as they take on roles, let their voices flow; show off their bodies and talents. I also ask people to draw their visions of an addiction-free life and/or their future without self-abuse. In 30 minutes we usually have a wonderful array of brightly coloured drawings – which each person explains with glowing pride.

'PUT DOWNS'

We have probably all been 'put down' by adults, brothers and sisters or teachers at some time, for 'showing off'. Unfortunately, this can leave deep scars on your creativity, and even completely repress it. If you watch young children, they get so excited about everything they produce – from a 'poo' in a potty to colourful paint splodges on paper. Human beings of all ages, with a little encouragement, can experience great excitement and power from the act of creation. First there's nothing but emptiness, space. Then, through the drawing together of different parts of yourself (and how you interact with the world), there is something real, tangible, existing independently from you. Something to be proud of, so you can say 'look what I've done' with pride and satisfaction. Unfortunately, because most of us get 'put down' for being 'bigheaded' and 'boasting', our creativity can get stunted for years. We are supposed to be humble, modest, meek about our productions. Yet each act of creation is an act of creating yourself anew, a rebirth, an expression of who you are. Your creative expression should be welcomed, trumpeted, cooed over, treasured (just as you should have been as a baby).

GIVING YOURSELF PERMISSION

All I do at workshops is give people permission to be creative – permission to be themselves. All that gets in the way usually is fear. Fear of not being good enough, and therefore being humiliated, or being too good (and being hated for being good). People feel competitive, defensive, hard on themselves for not being perfect. But we all have a real need for being creative, and if you can identify and meet that need for yourself, you are on your way to a fulfilling, addiction-free life.

As you give up your addictions, work through the feelings and begin to build yourself anew – you may find yourself opening up to the beauty of flowers, the countryside, the sea, music and many other forms of creative art in a way you never have before. The healing process sensitizes you to 'benign reality' – that is, all that is good, inspiring, beautiful in the world. As people throw off their addictive shackles, they suddenly find joy in children, excitement in colours, sensual pleasure in good, wholesome food. All you have to do is give yourself permission to have all that is good and beautiful in your life. And giving yourself permission is based on believing you are worth it – as indeed you are.

BEAUTY AND ORDER

If you go to someone's home and it is dirty, untidy, unattractive, and uncomfortable, it will tell you a great deal about how they really feel about themselves inside. It doesn't take a lot of money or a diploma in interior design to make your home environment pleasant. But it does need you to decide that you deserve beauty and order in your life. Sometimes clients reveal to me a great deal of despair over this aspect of their lives. They feel helpless about the mounds of (untouched) paperwork, piles of ironing, peeling paint, heaped up dirty dishes and films of dust on every surface. They feel overwhelmed about where to start changing things. Often, all that is needed is a roll of black plastic bags and a friend's encouraging support while they empty drawers and cupboards of detritus.

If your life is full of addictions, then it doesn't really matter what your environment is like, because you are inured to it. But when you start to get off the hook, you may well feel an urge to 'spring clean' yourself and your home.

It is not being 'vain' or 'too houseproud' to make ourselves and our homes beautiful, or at least comfortable. 'Beautifying' doesn't mean having plastic surgery or redecorating your house, but rather describes an atmosphere. If you want peace and tranquillity, if you want to feel good about yourself both inside and out, it will take a little time, thought and investment of your resources, to create beauty and order.

This is not the same as saying you've got to 'keep up with the Joneses' and have all the latest hi-fi equipment, a landscaped garden, and a wardrobe full of designer clothes. It means basing your life on a belief that your deserve good treatment, and indulging yourself and your senses accordingly.

Beautifying Yourself

Now it's time to make a personal assessment, once again recording your answers in your notebook.

1. How much time and thought do you spend on your appearance?

....

2. Do you always wear the same colour clothes?

....

3. Do you have a favourite outfit? If so, what is it like – and why do you particularly like it?

....

4. What do you do, to look after your body and general appearance?

....

5. How do you pamper yourself?

....

6. Is there anything more you would like to do to beautify yourself?

....

Beautifying Your Home

1. How much time and thought do you spend on your home?

....

2. What do you do to look after your home?

....

3. How do you make your home welcoming, comfortable, pleasant?

....

4. Is there anything more you'd like to do to beautify your home?

....

What do your answers reveal about your attitude to yourself and your home? Can you see any other ways you might give yourself and your home more loving attention?

EVERYDAY CREATIVITY

Creativity is essential to our well-being as human beings. Apart from creating your own image and your home environment, how else do you use your creativity in your everyday life? You may not have thought of the following activities as being creative, but they are.

- Cooking. Creating meals and using colour, texture, aromas, tastes.

- Making things – from clothes to bookshelves. This uses your intellectual, manual, conceptual and visual skills, creatively.

- Wrapping presents. A creative task, using colour, ribbon, paper, glitter, bows.

- Gardening. Planting window-boxes, flower pots, rockeries, vegetable patches, flower beds. Using colour, textures, scents, and your manual, visual, conceptual skills.

- Playing with children – and following their play. Using your creative imagination and entering into their world. You can be in a wonderland, fighting star wars, on incredible journeys, having a picnic, using toys, paints, paper, games, fabrics, videos, play dough, balls, string, building bricks, cushions, sheets.

- Singing. From singing 'happy birthday to you', to yourself in the bath or shower, singing along with the radio, or to children to get them to sleep. Using your voice creatively, in these and many other ways.

- Dancing – around your living room, at a party, at a disco.

- Learning to waltz at a local evening class, or Greek dancing while on holiday. Using your whole body creatively.

- Speaking languages. Playing with words, learning new dialects. If your speak more than one language, luxuriate in your ability to communicate creatively, learn a new language and use your vocal and conceptual powers to the full. Learn sign language – which includes your visual and manual skills and enables you to speak without sound.

- Writing letters, diaries, notes, cards. We seldom count this as writing, but it is very creative and you use your creative imagination to communicate your experiences and ideas.

- Work. We are creative all the time. We have ideas, communicate and agree them and then put them into practice, we problem-solve, do practical things, from window-dressing to house-building or creating office systems. Your work probably takes up a large amount of your creative energy.

We seldom acknowledge the above as creative activities, but they all are. We just take them for granted. Yet, people are keen to 'show off' their neatly weeded gardens, freshly decorated kitchens, new clothes and haircuts, their successes at work as a sign of themselves. After all, anything that improves our environment is worth encouraging. Bringing your creativity to bear on yourself, your surroundings and your everyday life is meeting a real need and therefore can be deeply satisfying.

CREATING ART

Many of us are frustrated artists and, as a consequence, think 'Art' is the preserve of the rich, the insane, the hugely talented, the warped, or all four. Yet, artistic endeavour is a necessary way of life for many people who are striving to draw out this deepest form of creativity from within themselves. The idea that everyone has a book inside them struggling to get out is often ridiculed, but there is something in this. Art, or the creation of something original, out of you, your experience, your environment, your language, your perspective, your creativity, is an expression of you. It is usually only possible to do this once you believe you have something to communicate, so first you need some degree of self-esteem.

It may be you need a way to vent your emotional pain in order to heal. And the process of creating art can also be the way to heal pain, whether you realize it or not. That is why drama, music, painting are often used as therapies to heal people who have suffered mental or physical distress. Tapping creative energy can be a profoundly effective way of healing deep-seated hurts. It is also a process which, in itself, is deeply nourishing and pleasurable, and which far too many people deny themselves.

Make Space to Create

To be able to create art, you have to allow yourself time and space. You need to think you are worth the effort, that you deserve to 'have a go'. Many writers, painters, sculptors, musicians, photographers, dancers have to battle with themselves to make the space to create. You have to be able to go into the deepest parts of yourself and face who you really are, to create. It can make you feel very vulnerable and afraid that there'll be nothing in there when you look for it, or that what you create will be 'bad' or 'worthless'. This feeling tends to reflect how you are probably feeling about yourself anyway. But success breeds success, and the more you can appreciate and value what you create, the more your creative powers will evolve. So be assured that you can improve – everyone always can – but allow yourself to be at the level you are now, in order to make a start. Then be willing to learn, to explore, to grow. To do so is both courageous and very rewarding.

HOW TO MEET YOUR CREATIVE NEEDS

The idea that artists are born, and not made, is very off-putting to people starting out. It also feeds an illusion that artistic endeavour is the preserve of an elite, reserved for the few blessed with genius. And, of course, in every creative sphere there have always been creative talents amounting to genius. But most art (even by those of genius) is the product of:

- Extremely hard work. You just have to practise your art over and over and over, and over again. It requires dedication, determination, a desire to create your particular vision and be willing to fail many times in the attempt.

- A willingness to learn. No-one knows everything when they start creating art. Many artists have gone to their local adult education institute for evening classes, or on courses and workshops designed to bring out their talent. There is nothing shameful about needing help to open yourself up artistically – the only question is whether you're willing to make the effort it takes, and especially be willing to learn.

- Following your passion. Your passion, your fire, your desire to make art creates energy. If you can let yourself follow what excites you and set aside all the 'shoulds' and 'oughts' and censors in your head that criticize and constrain, you can let yourself fly and enjoy every absorbing minute.

You may already be embarked on an artistic career, such as being an actor or graphic artist, in which case you will probably need to keep going in your sphere, gather confidence about your existing skills and develop new ones. You may also want to supplement your existing artistic work with something different, but related, for relaxation.

So follow whatever creative form excites you, let yourself explore and experience all sorts of artistic pursuits. You may want to do them alone or go on specialist workshops, or courses to get feedback from other people. These activities can include:

- Music. Singing, playing instruments, writing songs, dancing, drumming, humming, recording yourself, joining a choir, setting up a band.

- Visual arts. Painting, drawing, sculpture, photography, video-making, graphic art, ceramics.

- Performance. Acting, singing, dancing, poetry, mime, broadcasting, street theatre.

- Writing. Poetry, prose, newsletter articles, plays, scripts for TV and radio.

- Editing, producing and directing. Plays, newsletters, magazines, TV and radio programmes, and films.

- Design. Fashion, furniture, household goods, buildings.

The above is by no means exhaustive, and you may think of many others.

LET YOURSELF GO

Don't be put off by thinking you're not 'great'. Don't be disheartened if you are not a Madonna, a Monteverdi or a Milton straight off. Don't get caught up in competition and self-criticism, that's just a negative downhill path. Enjoy yourself; be positive. Many artists feel the process of creation is much more enjoyable and important than the ultimate product. It is like a kind of giving birth – *to yourself*. Conceiving, bearing, nurturing and then giving birth to your artistic progeny is the essence of being alive. So allow yourself the joy of meeting your creative needs, stop waiting, give yourself permission to make a start; have fun and revel in everything that brings passion, light and fulfilment into your life.

LET YOURSELF GO and overcome your addictions.

Chapter 15

━■○■━

Meeting Your Intellectual Needs

We seldom pay direct attention to meeting our intellectual needs, but being adequately mentally stimulated is an important part of life. So, if you don't know how to meet your intellectual needs (or even know what they are), you can suffer a great deal of boredom. Whether you have been to University or not, and/or followed any further or higher education, you will probably have intellectual needs that have still to be satisfied. And learning to use your mind to its fullest potential can be very exciting and rewarding.

WHAT ARE YOUR INTELLECTUAL NEEDS?

Answer the following questions in your notebook to get a clear idea what your needs are.

1. What do you think your intellectual needs are?

   ....

2. How do you meet them at present?

   ....

3. How would you like to develop your intellectual needs further?

....

Keep your answers in mind while reading the rest of this chapter.

CONQUERING BOREDOM

When you give up your addictions you can feel extremely bored, dissatisfied, and restless. Time seems to hang very heavily. You may try to distract yourself from thinking and feeling too much, because your emotions are surfacing and feel very raw. This is when video and computer games, and perhaps gambling, can be so attractive. Not only because of the emotional excitement and adrenalin buzz to be gained from risk and competition, but because of the *intellectual* challenge of pitting your wits against a system.

Conquering boredom is a necessary part of getting off the hook. You will feel more and will need to learn how to accept, release and live with these feelings. Boredom is often a major reason for people getting addicted in the first place, and underlying the boredom usually there is a pool of chronic isolation, disconnection, fear and anger. So when we get off the Addictive Treadmill, by giving up the addictions that, albeit temporarily, used to blunt such feelings, facing them can be daunting.

But you can conquer boredom – and it will be necessary to do so if you want to stay off. Learning how to meet your intellectual needs, and conquer boredom, is the ultimate challenge: you can't rely on someone or something else to amuse you – you have to do it for yourself. It is therefore very empowering, to decide what you need for yourself intellectually, and then set about getting that need filled.

BUILDING YOUR INTELLECTUAL SELF-ESTEEM

Most of us feel stupid to some extent, and this lowers our self-esteem. This feeling usually stems from how we were treated at school while learning, how well we 'competed' with brothers and sisters and schoolmates, whether we got 'put down' for our social class, skin colour, gender, physical ability, culture. We also are made to feel unintelligent because of how we've fared in tests and exams, although these usually only measure how good we are at jumping through those particular academic hoops. Yet, we all need mental stimulation, whether we think we're intelligent or stupid. To keep thinking, learning, and exchanging information with other people about particular subjects and ideas, is a PLEASURE.

So whether you think you're 'an intellectual' (that is someone who spends a lot of time reading, and thinking about theories and ideas) or not, you will have intellectual needs. Throw off the term 'stupid', if it has been applied to you, and start building your self-esteem instead. Notice your intellectual achievements so far, take pride in what you do know, rather than brood over what you don't. It is a fact that, whatever age you are and whatever educational and ability level you have achieved to date, it's never too late to start developing your mind.

Emotional Blocks

You may well have some emotional blocks to understanding certain subjects. You may feel daunted by theory of Quantum Mechanics, baffled by learning German or infuriated by Existentialism (so many of us are). This doesn't mean you *can't* understand these things if you really want to. It usually means you feel emotionally blocked about understanding them. You may well need to cry, shout, rage, have a 'tantrum' while trying to learn. The feeling of frustration can be released if you pinpoint how you actually feel. You don't need to be defeated by any subject – but you may have to work at freeing up your intelligence to be able to think clearly. If you re-read Chapter 10: Meeting Your Emotional Needs, this may help you to deal with your feelings.

It can be very frustrating not to understand something, and that feeling of frustration may well go back to earlier learning experiences where you were made to feel stupid. We have all sat in classrooms, in front of teachers, or been lectured by parents, or tried to follow TV programmes on subjects we don't understand. At least some of the time that will have been because whoever was lecturing us wasn't a very inspiring teacher.

The feeling of confusion is usually an old chronic distress. As young people (and as adults) we may need to be able to ask many questions in order to understand something. Of course, different people have different aptitudes, but we are usually 'shut up' before we can ask all the necessary questions we need for learning. Classroom teaching necessarily has to go at a pace which suits the majority, so when we need a bit more time or explication to absorb information we get left behind, and those who catch on fast, get bored and frustrated.

We are often humiliated by people when we ask questions, because they sneer, 'You mean, you don't know that?' or, 'You're thick if you don't know the answer'. Our fear of being ridiculed like this can make intellectual equipment seize up.

You can't ask the TV questions either. It pours out information at a high rate and we sit there passively, trying to absorb what we can. TV can confuse more than clarify, and sometimes it even frightens us. So, deciding to remove any emotional blocks – by releasing feelings about past and present learning experiences – and becoming ACTIVE about learning, is the only way really to start meeting your intellectual needs.

Gender Stereotypes

Women sometimes feel certain subjects are male orientated, such as physics, car mechanics and engineering. Men can feel other subjects – cookery, languages, psychology – are female orientated. This is complete nonsense. Subjects don't have a 'gender' basis, but the way they are often taught does. Also, there are expectations on girls and boys to 'fit in' to our culture, with girls directed towards arts and boys towards science. This reinforces the stereotypes of girls being soft and arty, and boys being hard and mechanical.

In fact, girls can learn science, and boys can learn cookery – no problem. But they may have to be pretty determined and be prepared to undergo some painful haranguing from their peers and family, and overcome wider obstacles like exams and job interviews, in order to succeed.

How subjects are presented is also important. If they are taught drearily, at any level, people will find them hard to understand. But if courses are designed to engage people in learning and stimulate the imagination (and not just passing exams), then there is much more likelihood of stimulating the intellect.

MEETING YOUR INTELLECTUAL NEEDS

If you want to take charge of your own intellectual needs, try some of the following activities. Some you may carry out alone, others you may do along with people. Aim for a combination of the two, so that you do not become isolated in your intellectual pursuits.

Reading. This is an invaluable, inexpensive and readily available source of intellectual stimulation. It is a way of broadening your mind, learning, experiencing intense emotions, exploring the world, from the comfort of your armchair and at your own pace.

If you don't know where to start reading, make a list of all your favourite topics (travel, gardening, yoga) or types of writing (thrillers, romance, classics) and go to your local library and/or bookshop and ask if they can suggest some appropriate authors. Don't be shy about this. People who do this kind of work enjoy nothing better than to share their expertise. It is much more interesting for them than just stamping books or ringing up the cash till. Bigger bookshops in large cities and towns offer a greater choice, as do large reference libraries. Do you read fiction or non-fiction, or both? Dabble, experiment, try new types of writing.

Also ask your friends, work colleagues, family, children if they can recommend a good read. Women's and men's magazines usually have a book reviews page or column, and the 'quality' Daily and Sunday newspapers (such as the *Guardian*, the *Observer*, the *Independent On Sunday*), have extensive reviews of new books, articles on authors and trends in literature. Inform yourself. There are also radio programmes on Radio 4 and TV arts programmes which review books.

You could also join a local evening class, specializing in a particular subject or genre of writing (from Art to Zen Buddhism; Autobiography to Westerns). This will probably lead on to reading new authors, and communicating with a group of fellow students equally interested in your chosen subject.

You could also set up a reading group. Think of two or three people you know who like books and talking about reading. Suggest you meet once a month to discuss a particular book which you all read. This can be a very sociable event. Take it in turns to meet in each others' homes, and bring food and drink to share. Talk about what you liked, or didn't like about the books, thinking about the language, the plot, the characters, whether it was believable or not, engrossing or boring, what you learned, what you enjoyed. While exchanging impressions in this way, you will also deepen your relationships with the other people in the group. But avoid getting personal, if you disagree. Listen to what people say and respect your differences of opinion. Enjoy yourself.

One word of warning: If you know you are addicted to reading as a means of escaping reality and responsibility, then you may need to give it up, just like any other addiction, in order to deal with the underlying distresses. Perhaps you were a bookish child and fear intimacy with people? If this is so you may need a break from reading and, instead, it could be essential for you to branch out and meet other emotional, creative and/or physical needs instead.

Writing. This meets emotional, creative and intellectual needs all at the same time. You could keep a diary of your day, your thoughts, and experiences. You could also start writing fiction or non-fiction, or both.

There are many evening classes on the various forms of writing: technical, poetry, plays (for stage, TV, radio), screen-writing (for films, TV, etc), the novel, short story, and so on.

There are residential courses you can attend as a would-be writer. Look in *The Writer's Handbook*, (see 'Help' section) for further information. Also, a librarian in your local library and/or a large reference library will probably be able to tell you about such courses.

If you are serious about writing, there may be a local writers' group you can join, where you can read out your work in progress, and exchange constructive comments. You could always set one up of your own, by advertising in the local newspapers, and on your local library, bookshop and community centre notice boards. You need as few as three people to start – five or six is a good number. Meetings should last for about two to three hours, and everyone should get about the same amount of time in the group. Alternatively, if the meetings essentially have to be shorter, you can dedicate one meeting to each person's work, so there can be more of an in-depth discussion.

If you are unable to start writing, or are stuck, you can use a writing group to 'kick start' yourself. Just divide the time equally between members and take it in turns to write using the groups' attention as encouragement. You may feel shy at the thought, but having uncritical, uncompetitive attention while you write is especially helpful in getting over writer's block. This boosts confidence because you have something to show at the end of the meeting.

Further and Adult Education and Distance Learning. These are all very good ways of keeping the grey matter whirring. And some courses of Further or Adult Education lead to a

Diploma or Certificate, which gives you extra encouragement to stay with it. You might also want to do an Open University or correspondence course, usually known as 'Distance Learning'. These usually incorporate a week or more spent at a residential summer school, where you meet other students.

You might want to further your education on a purely academic level; or you might want to embark on a course which will enhance your job or career prospects. In this case, your employer (if you are working) might have a scheme whereby they can help you with course fees and give you special time off to go to college or sit exams. It is certainly always worth finding out if your desired course of study can be sponsored by your workplace.

Thinking time. We seldom pay much attention to the process of thinking, although it goes on all the time. A good idea is to set up 'thinking time' for yourself by getting together with a friend or colleague in order to 'think out loud' about something. It might be a problem that needs solving, or a course of action you need to think through, or you might be confused about something you're learning and need to talk about it, or you may need to 'brainstorm' ideas. Take it in turns to 'think' and 'listen' to each other. One person could talk out loud for, say, 15 minutes while the other person listens with attention (not commenting, asking questions or interrupting – simply paying interested attention). Then you could swop over, the talker now becoming the listener and vice versa.

It is amazing the difference it can make just to have another person's attention on you as you think out loud. It can help to get you 'unstuck', so you can clarify your own mind; and it stops you feeling so isolated. If you want to hear the other person's point of view about what you have been saying, ask them for what you need as precisely as you can. If you don't want advice or to hear their view because you want to puzzle it out for yourself, then don't invite them to tell you what they think, and stop them from telling you if they launch in regardless. You are the best judge of what makes sense to you. Trust your own thinking.

Problem-solving and general knowledge.   Again, this can be very intellectually stimulating and can take many different forms. You could do puzzles, acrostics, crosswords, word games of all sorts, which you can buy in newsagents, toy stores and bookshops. You can buy quiz books, quiz games, board games (such as chess or mahjong), and memory games which test general knowledge and fact-gathering.

You could try for membership of MENSA (see 'Help' section) which is a club for the highly intelligent, and meet similar people to yourself.

Some pubs now have 'quiz nights' which are hugely popular and a way of meeting like-minded local people. And of course, there are all sorts of TV quiz games, from *Countdown* to *Mastermind*. You might even want to volunteer to be a contestant, just for fun.

Some people make a career out of entering competitions on household products and in magazines, which tax their ability to think up 'jingles' and 'tiebreakers' and involve some general knowledge tests.

You can follow these kinds of pursuits alone, with friends, family and/or colleagues, and if you go to clubs and pubs, it can be a good way to meet your social needs, too.

Meeting your intellectual needs is an important step in your overall personal development. It can help build your self-esteem and an inner life, whereby boredom is conquered and the urge to hurt yourself through addictions, diminished. Also, you can accrue a store of information, interests and ideas which can make it easier to make new friends. But take care not to bore people with a monologue about your new-found knowledge. Nourishing your intellect is a very satisfying way of reclaiming your intelligence and putting you in charge of your intellectual life, while overcoming your addictions.

Chapter 16

Meeting Your
Spiritual Needs

Whether you are conscious of it or not, you have real spiritual needs which need to be met in order to overcome your addictions. In the broadest sense, 'spiritual' means emotions of a high and delicately refined nature relating to the human spirit and/or soul. As you begin to heal your emotional hurts by acknowledging, accepting and releasing them, you will probably find yourself increasingly able to love and be loved. You might even 'fall in love' for the first time. As your heart opens, your soul will begin to connect on a spiritual level with other living beings, with the beauty of nature, music, and art, all of which may or may not inspire a feeling that there's a 'Higher Power' of some sort at work in the universe.

Meeting your spiritual needs is an essential part of learning to be your own parent. It is important to take time to connect to yourself and others, to notice that you are part of the universe in all of its infinite complexity, to wonder at the magic of reproducing human and animal life, the ever-changing seasons, the laws of nature.

People sometimes begin to feel their spiritual needs while recovering from a painful crisis, such as a bereavement, a serious accident or illness, or being involved in a traumatic public event, such as a bombing or a major fire. The aftermath of these events usually prompts us to ask 'why me?'

We usually begin to think a lot about the 'big questions' of why we're here, what the world is for, how we got here, does God exist? while in our teens and early adulthood. Human beings have a deep desire to understand and connect with each other and the universe and these times of questioning can be deeply spiritual periods (which can recur many times throughout a lifetime), when we often withdraw into ourselves in a meditative way, looking for answers and listening to our inner voice.

THE POWER OF LOVE

A universal feature of things spiritual is the power of love to heal. Whether you go to church, chapel, synagogue or temple to follow a particular religion, or whether you believe in Shamanism, the laying on of hands in spiritual healing, or in forest fairies, or nothing in particular, you probably believe that love is a powerful healing tool. Most belief systems agree that there *is* power in positive energy, in doing good, in loving ourselves and others, and that negative energy (or 'evil') creates bad actions, especially when fuelled by hatred.

As long as human beings are in pain and feel unloved, unlovable, bitter, resentful, hard-done-by, and revengeful, then negative energy prevails. But as people begin to recover from past hurts, they also start to feel loved and lovable, they take interest in nature and animals, feel connected to their neighbourhood, town, city, nation and other people in the world. As you heal, you grow spiritually, freeing up your innermost thoughts, feelings and needs for deep connection.

HEALING POWER

There is a lot of pain and confusion in our culture about the power of religion. Some people feel very angry at what they feel is punitive 'mumbo-jumbo' doled out by particular belief systems. Others feel furious at what they feel is 'New Age' hocus-pocus. You may well have been brought up in a repressive atmosphere based on a particular religion and, quite rightly, feel suspicious and angry about even thinking of things spiritual.

You may feel political and/or pragmatic action is far more important and that going to church or meditating alone are real 'cop outs'. Indeed, when religions are used as vehicles for repression and destruction, it is really human distress abusing a particular belief system for its own selfish ends. Some cultures use religion as an excuse for enacting revenge and oppression, based on misinformation, prejudice and greed. This has nothing to do with spirituality; it is rather a continuation of human chronic distress. If spirituality is about channelling the power of the greater good and creating love in order to heal, it can have nothing to do with war, murder, pillage, rape and wanton destruction.

WHAT ARE YOUR SPIRITUAL NEEDS?

Take out your notebook again and write down your answers to the following questions, to clarify your own feelings right now:

1. Are you aware of your own spiritual needs? If so, what are they?
   ....

2. How do you meet them at present?
   ....

3. Is there any other way you would like to be exploring and/or meeting them?
   ....

MEETING YOUR OWN SPIRITUAL NEEDS

There are many ways you can meet your spiritual needs – and perhaps a variety of approaches will suit you. You may be clear about what you want, or you may be confused and need to experiment. That's fine, but whatever you do, be true to yourself. Also your spiritual needs are your business. You don't have to talk about them to anyone if you do not want to. Because there is so much confusion and pain in the world about things spiritual, you may find yourself attacked or ridiculed for holding particular beliefs. So it is often best to keep them to yourself and let them nourish you quietly.

Listening to your inner voice.   It is important to take time out to listen to your inner voice. Tune in with yourself on a walk in the country, sitting quietly in your room, in a religious building, such as a church or synagogue, in the bath and/or while doing yoga. Use silence to feel connected with yourself. Sometimes prayer and meditation provide the space we need for this. While we are connecting with a Higher Power, we are also connecting with ourselves. Trust your inner voice. Don't deny it. It may tell you really what you need to do, what course of action to follow, and if you trust it, you should be on the right track.

Some people feel frightened of silence, of being with themselves. But if you start with just five minutes a day, sitting comfortably, with your eyes closed, it will give you a wonderful sense of stillness and peace. Gradually increase the time you spend in this way, and you will begin to get in touch with yourself and be more centred, less torn this way and that.

Going to a place of worship or significant place.   Some people need to be in a place of worship to feel spiritual, perhaps sitting quietly or joining in a particular ceremony. Others find going to a significant place, such as Stonehenge, in Wiltshire, or the windswept Yorkshire Moors, is spiritually moving.

Connecting with nature. Some religions are based on nature worship, and many of us derive immense spiritual pleasure from looking at a sunset, standing on a cliff top looking over the sea, walking through a sun-dappled forest, or gardening. If you can feel connected to the glory of the natural world, if you experience a thrill when the vegetables and flowers you planted begin to flourish, you are connected to your spiritual self in everyday life.

Connecting with art. Some people feel deeply moved by paintings, drawings, buildings, music, dance, theatre, sculpture and every other form of artistic creativity. Some also feel spiritually moved by creating art themselves – whether this is by painting, lifting their voices in song, learning an instrument and making beautiful sounds, throwing pots, taking photographs, or making their own environment pleasing to the eye – all of these activities can fulfil a spiritual need for balance and harmony.

Connecting with children. The wonder of holding a new born baby in your arms, looking at the tiny fingers and toes, hearing the sweet, baby breaths, looking at fine, flawless skin: all these experiences can be deeply spiritual. Whether it is your progeny or not doesn't matter, we can all gain spiritual nourishment from being with babies, toddlers, small children, who are full of excitement, energy, wonder, originality, and of course, who expect to love and be loved. It is a truly amazing phenomenon that the human race can continually reproduce and love itself.

Connecting with animals. Some people experience a spiritual connection by working with animals or having pets. We may go to a zoo or travel the world and wonder at the variety of birds, mammals, and sea creatures. We may just have a domestic moggy or a goldfish, with whom we feel connected. When people begin to heal from their past hurts, they often begin to open up to animals as a first stage before beginning to connect with humans. Animals can feel less demanding, and therefore safer, than people. But the relationships between humans and animals are very significant, and the people who heal animals, like vets, or those who set up animal sanctuaries, are usually connected with the universe at a profound spiritual level.

Connecting with other human beings. Sometimes there are public events, such as political demonstrations, or disasters, like bomb attacks, when people get together to show their solidarity. The flowers left on the wire at Hillsborough stadium after so many soccer fans were fatally crushed, represented the love of complete strangers connecting with those who had died, and their families.

When people hold candles in the dark or hold hands round a nuclear base in protest, there is a feeling of commonality, of energy passed through the human chain, of love, hope and the possibility of the good overcoming the bad.

If you can feel sorrow at another human being's misfortune, not just because it reminds you of your own sorrows, but because you can empathize with the pain another experiences, then you are connected spiritually with the human race. We sometimes feel shy about expressing these feelings, but when people put their arms around complete strangers after a car crash or when a young person helps an elderly passenger off a bus, it is an act of connection, of giving, caring, loving, without any thought of recompense. Acts of kindness, selfless sacrifice, pity for another's pain, is what makes us spiritually connected.

Joining a group. You might want to join a like-minded group which will help you to meet your spiritual needs. Think about what you want, read the relevant theoretical literature and 'sacred' works, talk to people who are involved and perhaps go to several meetings before you commit yourself. Be sure that it is the right kind of organization for you. If you are pressurized in any way to make an immediate commitment it almost certainly is not.

A word of warning. Sometimes people get addicted to 'cults' like the Moonies or Dianetics because they are looking for parents and unconditional love. Some cults deliberately 'brainwash' people into feeling that there is only one way –

their way – of meeting your spiritual needs. Be wary of any organization that demands your 100 per cent loyalty, with no questioning or critical discussion, and particularly if they demand a high percentage of your income or personal sacrifice, such as cutting off totally from your family and friends.

Often, our 'frozen needs' for parenting and love can make these organizations seems very attractive because we finally feel cared for, contained and important. As we have seen in Part One of this book, we need to do the emotional work on our frozen needs, so that we can be freed up to identify and meet our real needs. No belief system, way of life, or religion is 'perfect' and believing in it uncritically will only damage you further. If you take the position of being your own parent, then no belief system or 'guru' can take on that role for you.

NURTURING YOUR SPIRITUAL LIFE

Your spiritual needs may simply be that you need to get out into the countryside more often and breathe the fresh air into your city-clogged soul. Or, it might mean taking your child to the sea-side and together revelling in the sand, sea and sky. It might be holding your loved-one tenderly in your arms and crying together about how much you care for each other. It might be putting your feet up and listening to a piece of organ music or jazz that makes you tingle all over. It might be going to church to pray, or chanting in front of your Buddhist altar. It might mean any of these things and much more. Whatever, it is crucial to nurture your inner, spiritual life as you move towards overcoming your addiction for the rest of your life.

Part Three

———●———

Staying Off
for Life

Chapter 17

━━━◉━━━

Staying Free

By now you have identified your addictions and decided to give them up. You might also have started meeting your real needs as Part Two of this book suggests. But the important question remains: how do you manage to stay off for the rest of your life? At 'giving up addictions' workshops I usually work with people making the decision to give up their addictions in front of the group. As we saw earlier, this usually brings profuse embarrassment, fear, and grief. People can think about giving up their addictions for an hour, a day, possibly even a week or, at a stretch, a month. But forever? That is usually too terrifying for words. A look of absolute horror descends when clients countenance never drinking wine, lighting up a cigarette or going out on a spending spree again.

HOW TO STAY OFF
FOR LIFE

As I've endeavoured to show in this book:

1. You need to identify where your addictions began, what function they have filled in your life so far, and why you have continued to let them control you.

2. You need to decide to take charge of your life, by giving up self-abuse (that is, addictions), learning to love yourself and building your self-esteem, so that chemical and emotional addictions become completely unattractive.

3. Instead of futilely trying to fill your 'frozen needs' for love, affection, nourishment, validation and security, you must decide to be your own parent. This means nurturing yourself instead of destroying yourself. And you can do this by identifying your real needs at the *present* time, for emotional, physical, sexual, social, creative, intellectual and spiritual fulfilment.

One Step at a Time

Of course, you can't do this all at once. You have to take one step at a time. It takes persistence, determination and commitment. It takes you believing you are worth the effort. It takes courage, because you will need to look at your life critically, and face upheaval and change. We can often be very impatient, wanting everything different right now, wanting all our problems solved this minute. We want immediate gratification, we can't wait (which is why addictions are so seductive because they promise instant solutions to long-term problems). Unfortunately (or fortunately), it will take time for you to go through the processes you need to go through in order to change your life. It will take the time it takes.

Your Turning Point

You will have to make the decision to stop hurting yourself, and you will probably only make that decision – wholeheartedly – once you can see YOU COULD HAVE A BETTER LIFE WITHOUT YOUR ADDICTION(S). Your turning point might even be down to feeling absolutely desperate – that moment when you can't bear to spend another minute on the Addictive Treadmill, and you know you've just got to get off – or you will die.

Whatever your turning point is, it is important to remember:

- Few people ever give up an addiction after just one attempt. But each time you try, you are continuing in the right direction – towards loving yourself completely.

- You can get there in the end, if you want to. There is nothing special about people who give up after one attempt; you can, too. It comes down to you believing you can; and you can.

- You can take it one minute, one step, one day at a time. You don't have to do it the hard way, and in total isolation.

- Willpower will get you so far, but you will need to do the emotional work necessary to stay off the hook. In fact, once you give up an addiction, your emotions will become more accessible, so it will be easier than you perhaps realize to get to the feelings. Remember: there is nothing really to fear about feelings. We are often more frightened of the fear, than of the feeling itself.

Backsliding

Inevitably people backslide when giving up addictions. Nothing is worse than having to pretend you have not just gobbled a Mars Bar, or three, when you have, although you are supposed to be on a diet or giving up chocolate. Sometimes we feel so bad about ourselves for backsliding, so guilty and full of self-loathing, that we punish ourselves even more. We eat more junk, or hurt ourselves in some other way.

Accept that you will probably backslide from time to time. It is only human. But instead of climbing on to a downward spiral of self-punishment, you could decide to give up your addiction yet again. You may need to make that decision over and over and over. And the next day, you may need to remake it again and again. That is OK. It doesn't really matter what you did yesterday. What matters is what you do right now. If you have always been the kind of person who punishes yourself for past bad deeds – give it up. You can take charge of your life. You deserve it. You don't need to beat yourself up for backsliding. Be gentle on yourself, forgive yourself. You are human and imperfect after all (thank goodness), and you can make a new decision, and remake it, in the very next moment.

Feelings Are Here for Life

Some people hope that once they have given up their addictions, and worked through the distresses underpinning them, that they will be free of feelings for the rest of their lives. Not so. Feelings are here to stay, they are here for life. Feelings are part of being human. Feelings of intense joy, of extreme pain, of despair, of happiness, will come and go according to what is going on in your life. What *can* change is your own attitude towards having feelings. If you can accept yourself as a fully feeling person, that emotional upheaval and change is entirely natural, that you feel what you feel because you're completely human, then you need not run away from feeling feelings – ever. If you want to become emotionally literate, you can. You can acknowledge when you feel sad or angry, or frustrated, and simply accept these feelings as part of being alive. You can give up fighting feelings, hiding them or pretending you haven't really got them. What a lot of energy goes into suppressing the truth, because we fear being humiliated by being open about what we want and how we feel. What a lot of time and resources go into people trying to puzzle out how to relate to each other.

A life without addiction is a life full of feeling, the whole spectrum – including joy. It's a life where you are fully alive, where you are not thrown by jealousy and envy. You can say, 'Yes, I feel jealous and envious, that must mean I want something someone else has got, or that I feel I'm missing out somewhere'. Life would be so much simpler if we were not afraid of showing who we really are – and a life without addiction can offer you that possibility.

Coping with Crises

You will have crises from time to time: problems at home, losing your job, having a miscarriage, rowing with a friend, experiencing stress, moving house, being in a car crash, separating from a sexual partner, having a child or parent die. Crises are part of life. As with feelings, crises are here to stay. What can change is your ability to handle them (and yourself). Instead of reaching for the whisky bottle, you can dive into someone's arms and sob your heart out. Instead of isolating yourself and being stoical, you can choose to confide in a good friend or seek professional counselling.

Becoming wise about yourself and your emotions means you can take control when times are hard. You can also choose whether or not you become involved in other peoples' crises. Maybe it is healthier for you not to do so, especially if you are a compulsive carer/codependent.

The key to living with crises is to expect them to happen occasionally, but not to spend every minute of every day anticipating the worst. If you can learn to trust yourself and others, then facing crises without addictive 'props' won't seem so daunting. Yes, you will probably feel a lot of uncomfortable feelings; there will be moments of confusion and pain. But that is all they are. You don't have to make a drama out of a crisis, especially if you are feeling more in charge of your life.

More Choices

If you decide to live addiction-free, you are actually deciding to give yourself more choices. You are no longer chained to the Addictive Treadmill. Your life is in your hands. You no longer crave relief through the 'feel good factor'. Instead, you can rest yourself, take exercise, communicate with people, treat yourself well.

Overcoming your addiction is a gradual process of steering your own life in the direction you want it to take. Not everything will always go according to plan – how could it? But if you deal with your fear of uncertainty, you can be much more flexible when multiple choices come your way. Living rigidly and stoically only leads to disappointment and isolation. Living flexibly brings much more satisfaction, power and freedom. At root, giving up and staying off is about loving and forgiving yourself, putting yourself first and taking charge of your life. No-one else can do this for you. Only you can do it. And you've got to want to do it – to do it.

POSITIVE LIVING

People always ask what they can replace their addictions with: 'How am I going to fill the time?' they ask. 'What will I do instead?' It is the old 'What do I do with the yawning gap?' conundrum. Well, first of all, you just have to feel the yawning gap. Recognize that it is there, and that it is very frightening. Secondly, you can adopt the attitude of being your own parent, which means you are in charge of your life and meeting your real needs. Thirdly, you can set your life on a new path, a path of living positively. Instead of looking for the problems, you can look for the challenges; instead of expecting failure, you can expect success. And it is to this positive perspective about how to live your life, that we turn finally.

Chapter 18

===◦===

Positive Living

The past is over. Whatever happened in the past has happened, but it doesn't need to determine the rest of your life. You can decide to step out and change. You can decide to put the past behind you and do something completely new – but you have to decide to be completely in charge of your life, and nobody else's – to do it. The only way you will finally kick your addictions, is by believing you are worth something. Up until now you have probably settled for very little. You have cut corners; you have accommodated people; you have put others first. From this moment on, all of that can change. You can base your life on what makes sense to you. You don't have to fit round other people's plans, or take their needs into account, before you work out what you want for yourself. You can take charge and live your life for you. You deserve it after all.

POSITIVE ATTITUDE

Everything in your life comes down to your attitude, and addictions hate positive attitudes because there's nothing for them to latch on to. You can have an attitude that nothing ever works out, that you deserve to be unhappy, that nobody likes you really, that you deserve not to be loved – and indeed, that may have been your experience. Or you can now decide that you deserve the best treatment out, that people like you (that you're totally lovable), and that you deserve the good things in life. A positive attitude will simply bring you more. Initially, you may feel that this is an unreal 'Pollyanna' perspective, that life simply isn't like that, and suffering in silence is more normal and even romantically attractive. But, it is true, that once you expect and want more, more will come into your life. You will attract more that is positive and good, so satisfaction lies just around the corner.

Building Your Self-Esteem

To get a positive attitude you have to keep building your self-esteem. For a start, why not count what's good in your life? It is so easy to dwell upon what is bad, and to continue putting your attention on what doesn't work, rather than look at what does. But *try* looking at what is good instead, and notice how well off you really are. Read the following and write down your responses in your notebook.

1. Think of three things that are going well in your life, particularly, things that you've made happen (such as getting a job, moving house, taking up a sport). Write them down.

....

2. Think of three things you like about yourself: in your work, your friendships, your everyday life, your appearance. Write down why you like these particular aspects.

....

3. Think of three things you know people like about you and you like about them. (Focusing on positive emotions in relationships is very important for building your self-esteem.) Write down the qualities you've singled out.

....

Now, why not try some of the following suggestions and see how they work for you:

Give up self-abuse.   Never again let yourself treat yourself badly. Don't punish yourself if things get hard, be easy on yourself. You only abuse yourself because you were abused in the past and believe it is a normal way of being. Don't push yourself when you are tired, don't kick yourself when you are down. Don't thrash yourself for being vulnerable. Don't hate yourself for having weaknesses. You are human after all, and that's fine.

Allow yourself to expand.   You may never have been to this place in yourself before, but you are allowed to grow bigger, to have everything you've ever wanted. You don't have to keep yourself small, manageable and needy to be approved of. You can approve of yourself right now. Give yourself slack to grow and expand beyond your wildest dreams.

Give up being rigid.   Rigidity comes from terror. It is a desire to control everything and be controlled. Giving up rigidity is scary because it means being flexible, and that can make you feel that your whole world is falling apart. Being flexible really means being able to think in the present, being able to change your mind if it makes sense, being able to say you were wrong when you were, being able to back-track when you need to. Being flexible, and giving up rigidity, means trusting you know what to do when you need to, and not having to cling to a ridiculous position just to prove, 'I'm right and you are wrong'.

Believe in yourself.   Nobody else can convince you that you are good or right. You have to believe in yourself, first and foremost, for your life to change. You can't wait for the perfect partner, a best friend, a great job, losing a stone in weight, or winning the pools. Life is flawed, nothing is ever perfect. Just believe that you are OK and on the right track, and take it from there. Nobody will ever be able to convince you that you are better than you feel you are – you won't believe them. In the end, you have to believe in yourself; nobody else can do that but you.

Love yourself completely. To stay off the hook forever, you have to love yourself in body, soul, spirit and mind. You have to give yourself the best treatment, think you deserve healthy relationships, decide you can have what is due to you. If you love yourself positively, you will eat and rest, and make time for yourself, exercise and take care of everything in your environment – because you're worth it. Nobody has to convince you, you don't have to impress. Simply, you are worth it. You are enough in yourself.

Forgive yourself totally. You have made mistakes, been silly sometimes, gone over the top, been churlish and unfriendly, hurt people. Yes, probably these and more. So what? You're human. And humans make mistakes. But are you going to base the rest of your life on getting things wrong? Would you expect the same impossible standards from anybody else, or would you forgive them? Can you forgive yourself? You should. You are worth it. Develop a positive attitude.

POSITIVE SUPPORT

Isolation is the root of all addiction. We can feel that nobody understands us, nobody really cares and that we have to fight our corner on our own. Isolation means retreating into ourselves, not believing that anyone is out there for us, and that everyone else has it easy. When you give up your addictions, for good, you necessarily have to give up isolation. This means looking around yourself and asking for help. This can be terrifying, especially if you have always done everything for yourself and don't believe other people are there for you. You may feel that other people could not cope with your needs, or that it is simply safer to meet them for yourself (or deny them altogether) because you don't want to risk being disappointed.

You will only stay free for good if you decide to give up your isolation – no matter how desirable it seems to hang on to it – if you ask for, seek out, even demand, continuing positive support.

Sources of Positive Support

First, look around you and see what positive sources of support are available to you.

- Look at your family. There is usually one member you can count on. Think about what you need from that person, and ask for it.

- Your friends. Maybe some are just acquaintances, others are bosom buddies. Look carefully. You may be discounting people who really care for you and want to help you. Give them a chance. Learn to take.

- Your partner, spouse, girl/boy friend, lover. He or she probably cares for you more than you realize. Give your partner/spouse/lover a chance to give their support by asking him or her for what you want. If that support is not forthcoming, then at least you know where you stand.

- Your colleagues/workmates. You can build pretty solid relationships with people you work with. Sometimes they can be more objective about your situation – and supportive – than people you live with or have simply known for a long time. Look around you at work. Is there someone you feel a connection with, someone who could be an ally?

- Workplace resources. There are sometimes very solid sources of support at work through personnel officers, administrative officers, even your boss. Sometimes formal or informal staff networks can be helpful, like women's groups, black workers' groups, trades unions, etc. You may have a company/office counsellor, nurse, occupational health visitor, whom you can confide in. Or maybe your workplace employs a counselling service, which offers confidential off-premises support? Look around. You may be surprised what is on offer to you, without any of it being recorded on your employment records. And if you are trying to give up cigarettes, alcohol or drugs, your workplace might even pay for you to go on a scheme, and/or offer time off, without reducing your holiday entitlement. Be bold. Asking for support may well pay off better than you could possibly imagine. And you don't need to feel ashamed; you are in the same boat as thousands of others.

- Organizations like the Samaritans, Alcoholics Anonymous (see 'Help' section for addresses and phone numbers), can offer immense confidential and personal support. There is a lot of help out there, just waiting to be used. It is not shameful to ask for help. It is *strong*. And asking for help is the first step in the right direction of living your addiction-free life for yourself – on your terms. You are not a helpless case if you phone the Samaritans. Many hundreds of thousands of people have done so before you, including counsellors, politicians, media people, artists, business people; in fact, anyone who has felt or feels overwhelmed by isolation at a particular moment with a particular problem.

- Specialist groups. There are self-help groups who deal with many addictive issues today, from alcoholism, to codependency, to gambling. Perhaps you need to join a group dealing with love addiction or maybe you need to talk to someone who has grown up in an alcoholic household, so need to contact Al-Anon or the National Association for Adult Children of Alcoholics (see 'Help' section). Whatever, you probably know yourself quite well, and if you are willing to begin to face the truth about your situation, you can get help from fellow survivors – which is often the greatest help there is – because they know just what it is really like being in your situation.

- Your GP, specialist clinics or health service may well be sympathetic if you explain what the problem is and what support you need. He or she can refer you on to specialist medical help which can be very supportive. If you fear you will be locked up in an institution if you talk to your doctor, get someone to go with you to the doctor's surgery, someone who understands your situation well and who wants to be an ally. You don't have to accept your GP's or any health professional's suggestions (unless you are a serious danger to yourself and others), so if you have any doubts, simply ask for more information, or time to think about any recommended form of treatment.

Write down what you want from your GP *before* you go, if you think you might go blank when you get there. You have every right to get national health treatment, don't cut yourself off from possible valuable sources of positive support.

To find out what other support is available, look in your local telephone directory and visit the social services department of your local authority. You can also look in local and national newspapers in the 'classified' or 'listings' section. You can also look on notice boards at your local library, and at your local community and/or health centre for local events/groups. Citizens Advice Bureaux usually know what's happening locally, so do call them up or drop in.

- Set up your own support group. If you cannot find the precise support group you want or need, setting up one yourself may be the answer, especially if you live in an isolated or rural community, or going out is quite limited for you. It may also cost less, because you don't have to pay a professional fee (as with private counsellors and therapists). It may also help you mix with people you feel comfortable with.

HOW TO SET UP A SUPPORT GROUP

First, look around you. Do you have friends, colleagues, acquaintances, family members, who are struggling with a similar addiction to yours? If not, you could advertise in your local or national newspapers, community centres, sports clubs, and you can use a PO box number (ask at your local Post Office), if you feel shy or nervous about giving your address and telephone number. You could also try advertising on your local radio station, again using a PO box number.

What to Look for in Support Group Members

- A desire to look at the subject seriously for themselves.

- An ability to listen to others, and not to interrupt frequently or judge harshly.

- A willingness to be open and honest (at least to try to be).

- Reliability. Willing to come to meetings regularly, and do what they say they will do is important.

- Punctuality. Arriving on time creates safety for everyone. Someone who is always late can be disruptive. You don't have to stand for it, but you do have to be firm.

- Lack of melodrama. Some people use groups to get as much attention for themselves as possible. Watch out for 'drama queens'. Be firm, but tactful, saying something like, 'I'm not sure this group is exactly what you want. I'd like some time to think about group membership'.

Size. A support group can be a minimum of three, a maximum of five or six. The bigger it gets, the more unworkable it becomes as members then get little time for themselves.

Gender. You may want your support group to be single or mixed gender, according to how 'safe' you feel. For instance, if it is a group about 'sex addiction', you may well want to make it all women or all men, or all bisexuals. Or, if it is a 'giving up smoking' group you may want a mix of men and women. Be clear about what you want, and why.

Simply ask each prospective member if they would be willing to come along for a preliminary talk with you for half an hour. Say this will give you both an opportunity to see whether you could work well together. If he or she agrees, make an appointment.

After these talks, think about each person you met. Close your eyes. Do you get a feeling of being 'uplifted' or 'dragged down' when you think of them? Do you feel any sense of their commitment, or do you feel they might be 'difficult' or 'hard work'? Trust your intuition and ask people to join only when you have thought about the group as a whole. Make sure there are talkers as well as listeners. Will some people be warm and others more reserved? Do you have a sense of commitment from the group as a whole?

Once you have decided which people you wish to have in the group, ask them to commit themselves to meeting fortnightly or every three weeks, or monthly, initially, to see how things go. Say that at the third meeting, you plan to have a review session so everyone gets to say how it is going for them. At this point, you can decide whether to continue as a group, to extend or dissolve it, continue as you are for three more sessions or six months, or whatever.

Venues. It is a good idea to have those first three meetings in your own home. Then, if you continue, rotate meeting in a different member's home each time, preferably in a room where you won't be interrupted or distracted. If at all possible, get away from a ringing telephone. If the person whose house it is has children, help them think about their child care needs, so they're not isolated with the responsibility – but encourage them to come to the group regardless. If they have child-care difficulties, it may be a good idea to suggest meeting there each time, so they can attend with the least amount of difficulty – especially if they are the single parents and/or the only parents in your support group (or you could club together and pay for a babysitter). If there is more than one parent in the group help them negotiate their needs, taking into account other child-carers available, age of children, income etc.

Lead the group. Don't be diffident about this, because it's always a good idea for any group to have a leader, and it might as well be you. A group leader's job is to make sure everyone gets to speak some time during the meeting and that no-one is left out or attacked. It is also important that at the end of each meeting the time and place of the next one is agreed.

How to Run a Support Group

There are innumerable ways to run a support group, but here are some helpful tips. No doubt once your group becomes established you will have plenty of ideas of your own.

- Start on time. Ask people to come on time and start promptly. This will show that you mean business. Don't wait until the last person has drifted in, because if you do you then give them power to disrupt the group. Respect the people who made the effort to get there on time.

- Allow two to three hours per meeting, with perhaps two short breaks for going to the loo, making hot drinks, etc.

- Whatever the group's agenda, it should be agreed at the outset that none of you will drink alcohol, take drugs or smoke during a meeting. Preferably, also, people should come sober and drug-free, so that you are all feeling reasonably fresh and attentive, and able to contribute positively to the meeting.

- Set a positive tone yourself. Welcome people and ask them to introduce themselves in turn, stating their name, why they've come and what they want to get out of the meeting. Ask them to say three things that they have enjoyed recently and/or that are going well in their lives (no matter how trivial). This should get the meeting off to a good start.

- Confidentiality. Ask group members to agree to being confidential to provide safety. Ask them not to chat with people outside the group about what was said within it, no matter how sorely tempted. **Confidentiality** is crucial to making the group work. Be sensitive to one another. When people bare their souls they can feel very vulnerable. Do not betray their trust.

- Take turns talking. It is a good idea to divide up the time in the group so that everyone gets the same amount. This gets round the problem of 'wordy' people who talk a lot and gives the 'quiet ones' encouragement to speak. You can use a timer or alarm clock, or simply look at a watch, to keep a check on the time. Suggest a member to time the first person's talking time, then rotate the timing responsibility by passing the watch round as the next person takes their turn. People can feel very relieved to know that they will all get equal time talking, even if they feel embarrassed at the thought initially.

- Handling feelings. It's fine for people to show their feelings during group time. In fact, talking may well lead them into feeling sad, angry, exhausted, isolated – or any number of mixed feelings. Don't rush in to shut them up or comfort them. Let them talk/feel unrestrained. If, however, they show real distress and you feel a word of encouragement or an arm around a shoulder or held hand would help them to let go, then do so, but gently. Let them know you are there and you care, but never interrupt and never distract. Released feelings is an essential part of the healing process. And for members of a group to know they can do so and be understood in a supportive atmosphere can work wonders and change their lives.

- Handling group conflict. Inevitably, most groups have conflict between individuals from time to time. Nobody can get on all the time. However, you have met for a purpose: to share support in giving up your particular addiction and staying off for good. The group is not about embarking upon an in-depth psychoanalysis. Try to keep people to the point, and not get side-tracked. However, you don't have to avoid all conflict, as it can be very fruitful in opening up issues for the group as a whole. If any members decide to leave, get them to talk to you about it, if they will. But don't try to persuade them to stay beyond the first three sessions. Nor should you go into in-depth post-mortems after they've gone. Keep focused on the job in hand – which is mutual support by the remaining members as you each work at giving up your addictions.

- Set realistic goals. Each member needs to set his or her own goals for the time until the next meeting. It can be something very simple – like not eating or drinking something specific, or going swimming once, or making one useful phone-call. Ask each person to write down their goal/s and take them away (the group leader should also make a note of all of them). At the next meeting, ask how the goals have gone, but don't guilt-trip people. Realistic goal-setting is very important and gives each person a chance to act powerfully and to help themselves get off and stay off progressively.

- Telephone support. You can feel at your lowest ebb at two in the morning and especially when everyone else is asleep or during the day when people are at work. One or more people in your group may have this problem. So find out what support each person needs and/or is willing and able to give. Some night owls will be delighted to be phoned at three a.m., while others would loathe it, but wouldn't mind being called at 8.00 a.m. During the day, telephone contact is invaluable for most people, as it breaks isolation. It lifts the burden if you can get to cry or moan for a while to a sympathetic listener. And one phone-call to another group member when you're wavering about backsliding can be worth its weight in gold, turning a 'Maybe I will give in to the urge,' into a 'No, I will stick to my decision.' Sharing a problem is definitely a great way of releasing feelings. Encourage people to keep in contact by phone between meetings. However, if it doesn't suit someone, don't try to pressure them.

- End the meeting with a round where each person says what they enjoyed about the meeting, states their personal goal for between now and the next meeting, and shares what they are looking forward to during the next few days or weeks. This enables the group to end on a positive note as they record the time and venue of the next get-together in their diaries.

A POSITIVE LIFEPLAN

Once you have begun to develop a positive attitude and organized support to help you stay on track emotionally, then the next step is to look at your life and plan what you want to do with it. Are you just drifting along aimlessly? Or do you know where you are going? Are you satisfied that you are fulfilling your potential? Or have you given up on that score? If you don't know where you are going, feel frustrated and are underachieving, addictions can seem very attractive because they blot out reality. But if you are on course and enjoying what you do, then there is less frustration, less isolation, and you feel motivated to treat yourself well.

I have seen so many clients struggle with feeling powerless about their addictions, which, in turn, makes them feel powerless about every other area of their lives. But taking charge and giving up addictions brings more pride, energy and sense of purpose and if you've achieved in one area, then you begin to believe you can achieve in others. Once you learn to stay off your addiction you can develop a lifeplan, and have a sense that the sky's the limit. As indeed it is.

What is a Lifeplan?

A lifeplan comprises your short, medium and long-term goals for achievement in terms of your career, relationships, home, health, fitness, money, etcetera. Work out a realistic step-by-step programme of action, which you can review and revise regularly to keep yourself on track. Lifeplanning is about creating the sort of life you always wanted to live – but for real, and for you.

How to Start

You first need to find a fellow lifeplanner, someone who is a friend or colleague and who also wants to get their life on track. Someone who can listen, who is encouraging and whom you feel you can trust. Think about your friends. Does any one of them fit the bill? Ask if he or she would like to join you in an exciting project to get what you both want out of life. Few people will turn down such a chance.

You need to agree to meet for about two hours a week or possibly two hours every two weeks, according to how busy you both are. It's best to meet weekly if you can, because you get into a rhythm. You each have one hour, which can be taken in smaller chunks, such as four fifteen-minute sessions, or two thirty-minute sessions, alternating with one another throughout. You need to be quite strict about keeping time for each other for lifeplanning to work. Meet somewhere quiet, perhaps alternately at each other's home, or if you can't be undisturbed there meet in a quiet café, or sit in a park if the weather's fine. You need to be uninterrupted for the time you are together, so don't meet in a pub or over a meal and don't drink or take drugs, it's too distracting.

You will each need a notebook and pen and a watch or timer. Then here's what to do:

1. Take it in turns to listen to each other, the 'listener' making notes for the 'lifeplanner'. Each one of you, in turn, will 'think out loud' for, say thirty minutes, while your partner listens (without commenting, interrupting, advising, etc). After thirty minutes, swap roles.

2. Start off by making three lists:
   i. How you spend your time currently (work, leisure, relationships, going out, domestic chores, evening classes, shopping).
   ii. Whether it is paid or unpaid.
   iii. Your skills and experience.

3. Then think out loud about what you would really like to be doing with your life (don't censor yourself). A good idea is to imagine yourself at 90 years old, looking back and talking about what you did with your life. This will focus your mind on what you would really like to be doing, deep down.

4. Note down what you would really like to be doing in the long-term. This might be writing a book, re-training for a

new career, moving to another country, having children, leaving your marriage – I repeat: don't censor yourself.

5. Work out the short- and medium-term goals you need to achieve in order to reach your long-term goal. Don't give up if you feel it's too difficult at this stage. People always feel like this when they lifeplan.

6. Now set three very realistic steps you need to take to move towards meeting your short-term goals. Write these down and commit yourself to meeting all three before you next meet each other to lifeplan. If only having one goal is sensible, then do that. One is better than none.

7. Set the next meeting time and place.

8. Say something you enjoyed about meeting each other to lifeplan. This sends you both off on a positive note.

At the Next Meeting:

1. Start by reporting back on what is going well, what has been difficult, and anything else you need to say. Remember, this is for you – it is not to impress anyone else – so be honest.

2. Check on each other's goals. Did you do the three things? If not, what got in the way?

3. As lifeplanners, spend your time thinking out loud about what you need to do next and set your three short-term goals again before you finish. If one or two of your initial goals are still outstanding, just reiterate them, perhaps adding one new one.

4. Arrange telephone support if you'd like to phone each other between sessions.

5. Set the next meeting time and place.

Meetings Thereafter

Every so often, revise your medium and long-term goals according to how things change as you begin to meet your short-term goals. Notice how far you've come since you started lifeplanning. And remind yourself, whatever stage you have reached, that nobody can say you're indecisive and drifting through life now.

Lifeplanning enables you to make decisions about your life and move forward. It helps you to put yourself first and make things happen, which is the way to live positively. This ongoing process will move your life away from being buried in addiction and towards discovering and celebrating the real you.

POSITIVE HEALTH

If you are happier doing what you want with your life, your health will improve. Your immune system is boosted when you feel positive and fulfilled, just as it is depleted when you feel depressed, frightened and aimless. If you adopt a positive attitude to your health, it means you not only look after yourself when you get ill, but you look after yourself every day to prevent illness occurring.

If you need reminding what looking after yourself entails, re-read Chapter 11, and the notes you made in your notebook at that time.

POSITIVE PLEASURE

For a long time, you may have believed addictions to be your only real 'naughty, but nice' pleasures. But if you adopt a positive attitude to living, then you can enjoy positive pleasure. This means doing things for fun that aren't based on self-abusive addictions in any way.

Here is one idea for getting yourself started. Take a large envelope and write on the side 'My Positive Pleasure Trove'. Then get 20 plain postcards or file cards and write on each one something you love to do for pleasure, relaxation and fun. For instance, on one card you could write 'go swimming'. On a second write 'phone my best friend'. On a third write 'play my favourite cassette – specific track'. On a fourth, 'have a hot bubble bath', and so on. Keep adding more cards as you think of more things you like to do and/or discover new pleasures. They can be simple, inexpensive and locally-based.

When you get home from work, instead of pouring a gin and tonic, lighting a cigarette, or slumping in front of the TV, pull out a card from the bag and simply do whatever is written on it. Give yourself positive pleasure every day – you deserve it.

Some people feel they have to 'save up' their pleasures and keep them for a rainy day. A positive approach to life means allowing yourself pleasure every day, from the simplest act such as stroking your cat, or something energetic like playing badminton or a special treat like having a sauna and professional massage. A life built on pleasure and fun leaves no incentive or reason for destructive self-abuse through addiction. Positive pleasure means having good relationships, lots of play, personal power, joy and, of course, lots of love.

POSITIVE RESULTS

As I told you early on in this book, my own life has been transformed by overcoming my addictions. I'm happier, healthier, more fulfilled and have more fun than I ever thought was possible. I have better relationships and feel there's masses to look forward to. I have also been able to pass on what I have learned by helping many courageous people over the years. Here are some positive results, to encourage you on your way to an addiction-free future.

Pat Fisher, 50, Retired Picture Researcher

'I smoked for 30 years, 25 roll-ups a day, and I used to cough my way into the kitchen first thing each morning and keep coughing until I lit my first cigarette. I tried to give up many times, and once managed to do so for three years, but always ended up smoking again. I was offered early retirement and I really wanted to take it, but couldn't afford to as I was spending at least £45 a month on smoking.

'In desperation, I went to an "Off the Hook" workshop in April 1992, and from that day I haven't smoked. What helped was seeing that I had started smoking as an act of rebellion in a time of stress and that I could decide to give it up and treat myself better. I have felt my feelings more strongly, have cried buckets and felt a lot of fear. But my self-esteem has grown from my pride about giving up. My hair, eyes and complexion are clearer, and I no longer get palpitations. I feel incredibly relieved to be free of my emotional dependence on tobacco. I am now working out what the future holds, which although scary, is also full of hope.'

Joanna Walker, 45, Part-Time Administrator and Full-Time Mother/ Housewife

'I always said "yes" to everything and took on more and more responsibility at work, at home – everywhere, in fact. I didn't realize I was codependent until I went to an 'Overcoming Addictions' workshop. I was shocked, really shocked, when I saw how my life was destroying me. I decided to give up being a useful doormat and from that moment my life changed completely.

'Although I have often felt guilty, frightened, sometimes agonizing over every decision, I resigned from a very demanding and underpaid job, stopped volunteering for everything, started saying "no" and got my family to take more responsibility at home.

'I have learned to put me first: I have lost two stone, I am much more confident and I like myself more. I look back and think, "My God, I was bloody depressed." Fortunately, I've now learned how to be happy. I don't ever think I'm not entitled to what I want, and I don't spend money to "treat" myself any more. I am a different person, more powerful and positive. I've got a completely new lifeplan just for me.'

POSITIVE LIVING IN THE PRESENT

Of course, there will be tough times living without addiction, times when you backslide or mis-handle a crisis or feel you are back where you started. You won't be, of course, but it will *feel* like that sometimes. If you can accept the bad times are 'blips' and get yourself straight back on track again by being powerful about meeting your own real needs, then there's no need for despair. If you can also accept that you are an emotional human being, and learn to live with those emotions, you can have a great life. Being your own parent and meeting your own needs means you are in the driving seat, you are in charge, and you can get what you want.

Deciding to get off and stay off could be the single most important thing you ever do in your life, because it is a decision to love and forgive yourself, to put yourself first, to say 'I'm worth it' while allowing yourself all that's empowering and good by living positively in the present.

Part Four

Help

Where to Get Help

The following organizations provide help, information and helplines:

1. EVERYDAY ADDICTIONS

ALCOHOL

Accept
Addictions Community
  Centres for Education,
  Prevention and Treatment
724 Fulham Road
London SW6 5SE
Tel: 0207 371 7477

**Adult Children of
  Alcoholics**
For information send an SAE
  to:
PO Box 1576
London SW3 2XB
Tel: 01983 615483

Al-Anon
Family Groups UK and Eire
61 Great Dover Street
London SE1 4YF
Tel: 0207 403 0888 (24 hour
  helpline service)
Web: www.hexnet.co.uk/alanon
Email: alanonuk@aol.com

Alcoholics Anonymous (AA)
General Information (UK)
PO Box 1
Stonebow House
Stonebow
York YO1 7NJ
Tel: 01904 644026/7/8/9/10/
  11/12 (many lines)

AA
Regional Service Office
(London)
2nd Floor
3 Cynthia Street
London N1 9JE
Tel: 0207 833 0022
(10am–10pm daily)

Alcohol Concern
Information about alcohol
Waterbridge House
32–36 Loman Street
London SE1 0EE
Tel: 0207 928 7377
9am–5pm, Mon–Fri
Web: www.alcoholconcern.
org.uk/
Email: alccon@popmail.
dircon.co.uk

Drinkwise
National Helpline:
Freefone 0800 9178282
(9am–11pm, Mon–Fri;
6pm–11pm, Sat–Sun)

**Greater London Association
of Alcohol Services**
30–31 Great Sutton Street
London EC1V 0DX
Tel: 0207 253 6221
9.30–5.30, Mon–Fri
Fax: 0207 520 1627
Email: glaas@demon.co.uk

Healthwise
General information on
drink, drugs and AIDS
1st Floor
8 Mathew Street
Liverpool L2 6RE
Helplines: 0800 289061/
0800 3583456
9.30am–7pm, Mon–Fri
Tel: 0151 227 4150
Fax: 0151 227 4019
Email: admin@healthwise.
org.uk

**National Association for
Children of Alcoholics
(NACOA)**
PO Box 64
Fishponds
Bristol BS16 2UH
Helpline: 0800 289061
9.30am–7pm, Mon–Fri
Tel: 0117 924 8005 (admin)
Fax: 0117 942 2928
Email: nacoa@nacoa.demon.
co.uk
Web: www.nacoa@demon.
co.uk

Promis Recovery Centre
Help with alcohol and all
    compulsions
2A Pelham Street
London SW7 3HU
Helpline: freefone 0800 374318
Tel: 0207 584 6511 (24 hours)
Fax: 01304 841917
Email: robin@promis.co.uk
Web: www.ftech.net/~promis

**St. Joseph's Centre for
    Addiction**
Specializes in drink and drugs
    counselling/therapy
Holy Cross Hospital
Hindhead Road
Haslemere
Surrey GU27 1NQ
Tel: 01428 656517
    9am–5pm, Mon–Fri

CODEPENDENCY

**CODA (Codependents
  · Anonymous)**
Send SAE to:
Ashburham Community
    Centre
Tetcott Road
London SW10 0SH
Tel: 0207 376 8191
    (answerphone information)

Helpers Anonymous
For people with a compulsive
    helping tendency
Tel: 0207 584 7383
    9am–7pm, Mon–Fri

DRUGS

**CITA (Council for
    Involuntary Tranquilliser
    Addiction)**
For people addicted to
    prescription drugs like
    antidepressants and
    tranquillisers
Tel: 0151 949 0102

Families Anonymous
For families and friends of
    people with a drug problem
Tel: 0207 498 4680

Narcotics Anonymous
General information – send
    SAE to:
202 City Road
London EC1V 2PH
Helpline: 0207 730 0009
    (24 hours)
Tel: 0207 251 4007

National Drugs Helpline
Freefone: 0800 776600
    (24 hours)

Release
Information and help on
  legal/illegal drugs
388 Old Street
London EC1V 9LT
Tel: 0207 729 9904
  10am–6pm, Mon–Fri
Fax: 0207 729 2599
After 6pm: helpline 0207
  603 8654
Web: www.release.org.uk
Email: info@release.org.uk

**The Drugs and Alcohol
  Foundation**
Counselling, groups,
  workshops and advice
18 Dartmouth Street
London SW1H NBL
Tel: 0207 233 0400
  9.30am–5pm, Mon–Fri
Fax: 0207 233 0463

EATING DISORDERS

Eating Disorders Association
Information, advice,
  counselling, newsletter
Wensum House
1st Floor
103 Prince of Wales Road
Norwich
Norfolk NR1 1DW
Tel: 01603 621414
  9am–6.30pm, Mon–Fri
Fax: 01603 664915
Youthline (for under 18s)
  01603 765050 4pm–6pm,
  Mon–Fri
Email: eda@netcom.co.uk
Web: www.gurney.org.uk/eda/

Overeaters Anonymous
PO Box 19
Thetford
Machester
M32 9EB
Helpline: 07000 784985
  9am–10pm, Mon–Fri
Tel: 01426 984674 (recorded
  message with UK contacts)

**The Maisner Centre for
  Eating Disorders**
PO Box 464
Hove
East Sussex BN3 2BN
Tel: 01273 729818

GAMBLING

Gamblers Anonymous
PO Box 88
London SW10 0EU
Tel: 0207 384 3040
    7am–12pm, daily

Gamcare
One to one counselling
    (behavioural model)
Suite 1
Catherine House
25–27 Catherine Place
London SW1E 6DU
Helpline: 0845 6000 133
    10am–10pm, Mon–Fri
Tel: 0207 233 8988
Fax: 0207 233 8977
Email: director@gamcare.
    org.uk
Web: www.gamcare.org.uk

SEX AND LOVE

**Sex and Love Addicts
    Anonymous**
Church Hall
St Mary the Virgin
Evershot Street
NW1
Tel: 0208 442 0026
Meets every Monday at
    6.15pm, including Bank
    Holidays

SMOKING

**ASH (Action on Smoking
    and Health)**
Information/lobbying
16 Fitzharding Street
London W1H 9PL
Tel: 0207 224 0743
Web: www.ash.org.uk

Quitline
Victory House
170 Tottenham Court Road
London W1P 0HA
Quitline: Freefone 0800
    002200 12am–7pm,
    Mon–Fri
Tel: 0207 388 5775
Fax: 0207 388 5995

**Northern Ireland Smokers'
    Helpline**
Tel: 01232 663281

Scotland Smokers' Helpline
Tel: 0800 848484

Wales Smokers' Helpline
Tel: 0345 697500

2. EMOTIONAL HELP

Arbours Association
6 Church Lane
London N8 7BU
Tel: 0208 340 7646
　10am–5pm, Mon–Fri
Fax: 0208 341 5822
Email: arbours@compuserve.
　co.uk

**British Association for
　Counselling**
For a list of accredited UK
　counsellors write to:
1 Regent Place
Rugby CV21 2PJ
Tel: 01788 550899
Fax: 01788 562189
Email: bac@bac.co.uk
Web: www.counselling.co.uk

**British Association for
　Psychotherapists**
For a list of psychotherapists
　write to:
37 Mapesbury Road
London NW2 4HJ
Tel: 0208 452 9823

**MIND (National Association
　for Mental Health)**
15–19 Broadway
Stratford
London E15 4BQ
Tel: 0208 519 2122
Fax: 0208 522 1725
Email: contact@mind.org.uk
Web: www.mind.org.uk

Relate
Herbet Gray College
Little Church Street
Rugby CV21 3AP
Tel: 01788 573241
Fax: 01788 535007
Web: www.relate.org.uk

Samaritans
Tel: 0345 90 90 90
　24 hours a day
Email: admin@samaritans.
　org.uk

Women's Therapy Centre
10 Manor Gardens
London N7 6JS
Advice/Information line:
　0207 263 6200
　10am–12pm, 2pm–4pm,
　Mon–Fri; 6pm–8pm
　Thursday
Fax: 0207 281 7879

3. ALTERNATIVE HEALTH

British Acupuncture Council
Park House
206 Latimer Road
London W10 6RE
Tel: 0208 964 0222
Fax: 0208 964 0333
Email: info@acupuncture.
    org.uk
Web: www.acupuncture.org.uk

**General Council and
    Register of Naturopaths**
Send SAW and £2.50 for
    register
Goswell House
2 Goswell Road
Street
Somerset BA16 0JD
Tel: 01458 840072
Fax: 01458 840075
Email: admin@naturopathy-
    org.uk
Web: www.naturopathy.org.uk

**General Osteopathic
    Council**
Osteopathy House
176 Tower Bridge Road
London SE1 3LU
Tel: 0207 357 6655
Fax: 0207 357 0011
Email: gosc-uk@dial.pipex.
    com
Web: www.osteopathy.org.uk

Hale Clinic
7 Park Crescent
London W1N 3HE
Tel: 0207 637 3377
Fax: 0207 323 1693
Email:
    admin@haleclinic.com
Web: www.haleclinic.com

**Middle Piccadilly Natural
    Healing Centre**
Holwell
Sherbourne
Dorset DT9 5LW
Tel: 01963 23468
Fax: 01963 23764
Email: eheart@compuserve.
    com

Natural Federation of Spiritual Healers
Old Manor Farm Studio
Church Street
Sunbury-on-Thames
Middlesex TW16 6RG
Tel: 01932 783164
Fax: 01932 779648
Email: office@nfsh.org.uk
Web: www.nfsh.org.uk
Healer referral helpline: 0891 616080 (Premium rate call, Mon–Fri, 9am–5pm)

Neal's Yard Agency for Personal Development
BCM Neal's Yard
London WC1N 3XX
Tel/Fax: 07000 783704
Email: info@nealsyardagency. demon.co.uk

The Society of Teachers of the Alexander Technique
20 London House
266 Fulham road
London SW10 9EL
Tel: 0207 351 0828
Fax: 0207 352 1556
Email: office@stat.org.uk
Web: www.stat.org.uk

The Yoga for Health Foundation
Ickwell Bury
Ickwell Green
Biggleswade
Beds SG18 9EF
Tel: 01767 627271
Fax: 01767 627266

4. GENERAL HELP

DEPRESSION

Depressives Anonymous
Tel: 01482 860619
Helpline: 01702 433838
9am–9pm, 7 days a week

DISABILITY

RADAR
For information and advice
  for people with disabilities
Unit 12
City Forum
City Road
London EC1V 8AF
Tel: 0207 250 3222
  10am–4pm weekdays
Fax: 0207 250 0212
Minicom: 0207 250 4119
Email: radar@radar.org.uk
Web: www.radar.org.uk

MIND

MENSA

Mensa House
St John's Square
Wolverhampton WV2 4AH
Tel: 01902 772771
  8.30am–4.30pm, Mon–Fri
Fax: 01902 422327
Email: mensa@dial.pipex.com
Web: www.mensa.org.uk

GAY/LESBIAN

**London Lesbian and Gay
  Switchboard**
PO Box 7324
London N1 9QS
Helpline: 0207 837 7324
  (24 hour)
Web: www.llgs.org.uk

5. JOURNALS

Caduceus
Healing and new
  consciousness
38 Russell Terrace
Leamington Spa
Warwickshire CV31 1HE

Tel: 01926 451897
Fax: 01926 885565
Email: caduceus@oryx.
  demon.co.uk

6. BOOKSHOPS WITH BOOKS ON ADDICTION

(Mail order service available)

Compendium Books
234 Camden High Street
London NW1 8QS
Tel: 0207 267 1527
Fax: 0207 267 0193
Email: compbks@dircon.
  co.uk

Dillons
82 Gower Street
London WC1 6EQ
Tel: 0207 636 1577
Fax: 0207 580 7680
Email: orders@dillons.org.uk
Web: www.dillons.co.uk

Amazon.co.uk
Over 1.5 million titles, including up to 50% off UK bestsellers.
Fast delivery, easy searches. Web: www.amazon.co.uk

FURTHER READING

The following books are particularly helpful to read when recovering from addiction:

ALCOHOL
Sober and Staying That Way by Susan Powter (Simon & Schuster, £10.99)

You Can Free Yourself From Alcohol and Drugs by Doug Althauser (New Harbinger, £11.99)

DRUGS
Prozac Nation: Young and Depressed in America, a memoir by Elizabeth Wurtzel (Quartet, £8.00)

EATING DISORDERS
Fat is a Feminist Issue by Susie Orbach (Arrow, £6.99)

Fed Up and Hungry: Women, Oppression and Food by Marilyn Lawrence (Women's Press, £7.99)

The Anorexic Experience by Marilyn Lawrence (Women's Press, £4.95)

LOVE/SEX
Women Who Love Too Much by Robin Norwood (Arrow, £5.99)

Hot Monogamy: How To Achieve A More Intimate Relationship With Your Partner by Dr Patricia Love and Jo Robinson (Piatkus, £8.99)

MEDITATION/RELAXATION
The Three Minute Meditator: 30 Simple Ways To Relax and Unwind by David Harp with Nina Feldman (Piatkus, £8.99)

NUTRITION
Detox Yourself by Jane Scrivner (Piatkus, £6.99)

Fit For Life by Harvey and Marilyn Diamond (Bantam, £7.99)
The New Raw Energy by Leslie Kenton (Vermilion, £8.99)

PERSONAL GROWTH/THERAPY

Banished Knowledge: Facing Childhood Injuries by Alice Miller (Virago, £7.99)

Be Your Own Best Friend: How To Achieve Greater Self-Esteem, Health and Happiness by Louis Proto (Piatkus, £6.99)

A Complete Guide To Therapy: from Psychoanalysis to Behaviour Modification by Joel Kovel (Penguin, £7.95)

Detox Your Mind by Jane Scrivner (Piatkus, £6.99)

Dorothy Rowe's Guide To Life by Dorothy Rowe (HarperCollins, £7.99)

Emotional Intelligence: Why It Can Matter More Than IQ by Daniel Goleman (Bloomsbury, £7.99)

Feel The Fear And Do It Anyway by Susan Jeffers (Arrow, £6.99)

Homecoming: Reclaiming and Championing Your Inner Child by John Bradshaw (Piatkus, £10.99)

In Our Own Hands: A Book Of Self-Help Therapy by Sheila Ernst & Lucy Goodison (Women's Press, £8.99)

Self-Healing: Use Your Mind To Heal Your Body by Louis Proto (Piatkus, £7.99)

Strong At The Broken Places: Overcoming The Trauma of Childhood Abuse by Linda T Sanford (Virago, £8.99)

The Confidence To Be Yourself: How To Boost Your Self-Esteem by Dr Brian Roet (Piatkus, £8.99)

The Intimacy & Solitude Self-Therapy Book: Developing Inner Strength, Flexibility and Control by Stephanie Dowrick (Women's Press, £7.99)

The Successful Self: Freeing Our Hidden Inner Strengths by Dorothy Rowe (Harper Collins, £7.99)

You Can Heal Your Life by Louise L. Hay (Eden Grove Editions, £9.99)

RELATIONSHIPS
Codependency: How To Break Free And Live Your Own Life by David Stafford and Liz Hodgkinson (Piatkus, £7.99)

Dare To Connect: How To Create Confidence, Trust and Loving Relationships by Susan Jeffers (Piatkus, £5.99)

Facing Codependence: What it is, Where It Comes From, How it Sabotages Our Lives by Pia Mellody (Harper Collins, £8.99)

Families and How To Survive Them by Robin Skynner and John Cleese (Ebury, £6.99)

Life and How To Survive It by Robin Skynner and John Cleese (Ebury, £7.99)

Stop Arguing, Start Talking: The 10 Point Plan for Couples in Conflict by Susan Quilliam (Vermilion, £6.99)

The Good Relationship Guide: how to understand and improve male-female relationships by Dr Maryon Tysoe (Piatkus, £5.99)

Toxic Parents: Overcoming Their Hurtful Legacy and Reclaiming Your Life by Dr Susan Forward (Bantam, £6.99)

SELF-ABUSE
Woman and Self-Harm by Gerrilyn Smith, Dee Cox and Jacqui Saradjian (£7.99)

SMOKING
The Only Way To Stop Smoking by Alan Carr (Penguin, £8.99)

How To Stop Smoking and Stay Stopped For Good by Gillian Riley (Vermilion, £7.99)

Stop Smoking In 5 Days by Judy Perlmutter (Thorsons, £4.99)

Index